Series in Laboratory Medicine
Leo P. Cawley, M.D., Series Editor

Histopathology of the
Bone Marrow

Histopathology of the Bone Marrow

Arkadi M. Rywlin, M.D.

Director, Department of Pathology
and Laboratory Medicine, Mount
Sinai Medical Center of Greater
Miami, and Professor of Pathology,
the University of Miami School of
Medicine

Little, Brown and Company   Boston

To Hava and Danny

Preface

This volume is not a textbook of hematology, an atlas of bone marrow cytology, or a complete treatise on the pathology of the bone marrow. It is intended to encourage physicians interested in the morphology of the bone marrow to study histologic sections of bone marrow particles in addition to smears. A vast body of knowledge has resulted from the cytologic study of bone marrow smears. The examination of smears is extremely important; and the morphology of bone marrow elements as they appear in smears has been beautifully presented in many publications.

In some respects, however, the bone marrow has been a neglected stepchild of morphologists. At autopsy it is often disregarded because cytologic detail is obscured by autolysis, sawing artifacts, and decalcification. Also, special stains are often inadequate on decalcified tissues. Clinical studies of bone marrow have relied primarily on smears because of the technical complexities of preparing histologic sections and the lack of expertise in interpreting them. The bone marrow is the only organ in the body that has been studied primarily by cytology. Histologic sections add another dimension to the interpretation of bone marrow specimens and should always be examined in addition to smears.

This book presents a simple technic for obtaining sections and smears of aspirated bone marrow particles. The same technic has contributed greatly to the evaluation of bone marrow findings at autopsy. I also describe an approach to the interpretation of the bone marrow emphasizing primarily the findings in histologic sections. The chapters are arranged in the same sequence as the bone marrow report.

The emphasis in this book is on what can be seen better in sections than in smears. This includes the recognition of metastatic tumor cells and malignant lymphomas and the evaluation of cellularity, hemosiderin stores, and stromal changes such as serous atrophy of fat, vascular lesions, and granulomatous reactions.

The diagnosis of vascular lesions and granulomas in histologic sections of aspirated bone marrow particles extends the indications for bone marrow aspiration beyond the field of hematology. There is no question that bone marrow aspiration is a much safer and less expensive procedure than liver or muscle biopsy. Whether, in the diagnosis of granulomatous and vascular diseases, histologic examination of bone marrow particles will yield as many positive results as muscle and liver biopsies remains to be seen. Needle biopsies of the marrow make it possible to diagnose certain bone diseases, because they allow an examination of osseous trabeculae in addition to the marrow.

Arkadi M. Rywlin (Rivlin)

Acknowledgments

This monograph was written with the help of many people. Dr. Marvin Sackner, Chief of Medical Services at Mount Sinai Medical Center of Greater Miami, planted the idea of such a book in my mind. Dr. Carlos Dominguez, Chief of the Hematology Division at Mount Sinai Medical Center, as well as the attending hematologists, including Drs. Arnold Blaustein, the late Erwin Hoffman, Sherman Kaplan, Jacob Neber, Daniel Nixon, Simon Rozen, and Luis Wigoda, generously allowed me to process their bone marrows for my collection. My colleagues in the Department of Pathology and Laboratory Medicine, Drs. Beria Cabello, Jack Lubin, Rolando Ortega, Morton Robinson, and Maria Viamonte, made helpful suggestions and granted me the necessary time to work on the book.

William H. Atkinson, Charles Bailey, Christ Tavantzis, Klaus Juraschek, and Paul Showstark devotedly, expertly, and patiently photographed the slides. Mr. Theodore W. Eckels, President of Howmedica Inc., provided financial help for the publication of the color plates. Mrs. Patricia Pelicane did the artwork, and Elaine M. Abrams and Esther Ferguson spent many hours typing and retyping the manuscript.

The late Paul Marvan and James Roth, leaders of our histopathology section, processed the many bone marrow specimens with the loving care necessary to produce good histologic preparations. They also helped to compile the staining technics for the Appendix.

Jon Paul Davidson and Nancy Megley of Little, Brown and Company were very helpful, patient, and encouraging throughout the preparation and processing of the manuscript.

To all the named individuals and to many unnamed persons, mainly residents and fellows, who contributed to the bone marrow collection during their rotation through the department, I extend my sincere gratitude.

Contents

Histopathology of the
Bone Marrow

1 Bone Marrow Aspiration and Preparation of Specimens

General Principles of Bone Marrow Interpretation

A meaningful interpretation of bone marrow smears and sections requires familiarity with the clinical data. As a rule, the request for a bone marrow examination should be treated as a hematology consultation. Before the consultant—be he pathologist or clinician—aspirates the marrow, he must elicit the clinical history, perform a physical examination, and obtain laboratory data pertinent to the patient's problems. It is much more rewarding to view the bone marrow with this information at hand.

The first question the consultant should ask is why a bone marrow examination is desired. Was the request prompted by some abnormality in the peripheral blood involving the platelets, the red blood cells, or the white blood cells? Was the clinician attempting to stage a lymphoma, evaluating the status of the bone marrow during chemotherapy, looking for metastatic carcinoma cells, or working up a patient with a fever of unknown origin? It seems obvious that such basic information is essential, yet the pathologist often looks at bone marrow preparations sent to his laboratory with little knowledge of the clinical background. Objective morphologic findings can be reported in the absence of any clinical information, but such a practice is to be condemned. Not only does it prohibit the patient from reaping the full benefit of the depth of knowledge of the pathologist, but it also deprives the pathologist of the intellectual stimulation and invaluable experience gained from repeated clinicopathologic correlations. In the many instances when the bone marrow pattern is nonspecific, a consultant who is aware of the clinical problem can suggest additional investigations that may help establish a diagnosis.

A hematologic history should include racial and familial data, which are of importance in hemolytic anemias, storage diseases, and a variety of other hematologic syndromes. A dietary history such as strict vegetarianism might help elucidate a megaloblastic anemia. Information about prolonged or abundant menstrual blood losses may shed light on an iron deficiency anemia. Knowledge of drugs taken by a patient may establish a cause for thrombocytopenia, anemia, leukopenia, or aplasia of the bone marrow. Transfusions, vitamin B_{12}, and folic acid may change the appearance of the bone marrow and obscure the diagnosis. Exposure to toxins, use of alcohol, or excessive intake of cornstarch may explain certain bone marrow findings. These are just a few examples to illustrate the importance of the medical history in hematology.

Certain findings observed on physical examination are of interest to the interpreter of the bone marrow. Is there jaundice or purpura? Is the tongue smooth? Are the superficial lymph nodes diffusely enlarged or is there one mass of nodes? Are the liver and spleen enlarged? Is the bone tender to pressure? Are proprioception and the perception of vibration intact?

Significant laboratory data must be available at the time the bone marrow is interpreted. The hemoglobin, hematocrit, platelet, white bood cell, and differential counts should be known. The peripheral blood smear obtained at the same time as the marrow should accompany the bone marrow sections and smears. Other findings, such as blood urea nitrogen, serum protein, and hemoglobin electrophoresis, may help in the interpretation of the bone marrow.

Technic for Preparation of Bone Marrow Smears and Sections

Bone marrow for histologic and cytologic study may be obtained by incisional biopsy, needle biopsy, or needle aspiration. Bone marrow obtained by aspiration, when properly handled, yields excellent particles for the preparation of smears and sections.

The importance of studying histologic sections of bone marrow particles in addition to smears cannot be overemphasized [14]. Morphologic examination of the bone marrow, like that of any other organ, stands to gain from a combined histologic and cytologic approach. Stromal reactions of the bone marrow, granulomas, metastatic involvement, and vascular lesions can be appreciated much better in histologic sections than in smears. Unfortunately, many hematologists do not routinely examine sections of bone marrow particles, in part because of the relative complexity or tediousness of the described technics requiring anticoagulants, special equipment, or biopsy needles. The simple technic described herein, requiring no special equipment or anticoagulants at the bedside or in the laboratory, is intended to help popularize the histologic examination of bone marrow particles.

We use a simple method for processing aspirated bone marrow. The particles are concentrated without the use of anticoagulants or centrifugation technics. A nonincisional bone marrow needle biopsy is performed only when no material can be aspirated (dry tap), or when there is an indication to study bone histology in addition to the marrow.

Bone marrow aspiration can be performed at any site where the bone is superficial and easily accessible. The sternum at the level of the second intercostal space was used first [1]. The anterior superior iliac spine, the iliac crest, the posterior superior iliac spine, and the spinous processes of the lumbar vertebrae have all been recommended. When looking for metastatic carcinoma or multiple myeloma, it is of value to palpate the skeleton and to perform the aspiration in a tender or radiologically involved spot, provided that it is easily accessible.

Bone marrow aspiration, when properly performed, is a safe and harmless procedure. However, fatalities and complications have been associated with aspiration from the sternum. Bakir [2] described a death caused by cardiac tamponade from a laceration of the right ventricle following sternal marrow aspiration. Garnier et al. [8] reported a case of laceration of the intrapericardial aorta. A review of the literature by these authors revealed 15 fatal complications of sternal marrow aspiration. Of the 11 autopsied cases, 9 showed myocardial and 2 aortic lacerations. Undoubtedly, there are more unreported cases. I have autopsied a 34-year-old woman with sickle cell anemia who died of cardiac tamponade caused by a laceration of the right ventricle after a sternal marrow aspiration.

Rarely, a bone marrow needle may break while being inserted into the bone. An attempt should be made to clamp the distal portion of the needle with a hemostat. If this is not possible, the patient should be reassuringly notified of the mishap. The site of aspiration must be marked, a roentgenogram obtained, and a surgeon called in consultation.

Isolated pulmonary bone marrow emboli, apparently without clinical importance, have been described following sternal marrow aspiration [17] and also after the injection of contrast material into the marrow of the femur [9]. Growth of a sternal tumor mass following marrow aspiration has also been reported [7].

Hemorrhage may result from bone marrow aspiration from any site, but fortunately this condition is rare. We routinely apply a small pressure dressing following marrow aspiration. With this precaution, we have had no hemorrhagic complications even in thrombocytopenic and hemophilic patients. It is to be noted, however, that some authors consider hemophilia a contraindication to marrow aspiration [16]. In cases of a bleeding diathesis it is safer, particularly in obese patients, to perform marrow aspiration in the sternum, because it is easier to apply pressure for the control of bleeding.

Our preferred site for bone marrow aspiration in adults, as well as in children and infants, is the posterior superior iliac spine (Fig. 1-1). Aspiration at this spot is more comfortable for the patient and to a large extent avoids the pain and unpleasant sensation generated, particularly in the sternum, when the plunger of the syringe is pulled back. Also, to the best of our knowledge, no mortality or serious complications have been attributed to bone marrow aspiration from this site. The disadvantages of the posterior superior iliac spine, as compared to the sternum, are a thicker panniculus and a slightly less cellular marrow. In very obese patients, the sternum or spinous processes of lumbar vertebrae may be used for aspiration; however, with a long enough needle, the posterior superior iliac spine can always be reached.

The patient is reassured about the safety of the procedure; if he is overly anxious, a tranquilizer such as hydroxyzine is administered before the aspiration. The patient is asked to lie comfortably on one side. The operator locates the upper posterior superior iliac spine by a dimple in the skin which forms one of the lateral points of the rhomboid of

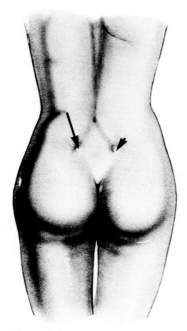

Figure 1-1
Rhomboid of Michaelis. The arrows indicate the posterior superior iliac spines, which form the lateral points of the rhomboid.

Michaelis (see Fig. 1-1). The skin overlying the spine is marked by an X made with the thumbnail and is swabbed with an antiseptic solution. We do not wear gloves for needle aspirations or biopsies of the bone marrow. In many years of experience, we have not had any infections. Careful washing of the hands and attention to common aseptic technics have proved adequate to prevent bacterial contamination. Because viral hepatitis can be transmitted by minute amounts of blood, the operator should not soil his hands with the patient's blood. We generally use lidocaine for local anesthesia; procaine and mepivacaine may also be employed. The patient should be queried about allergic reactions to these drugs. More patients are allergic to procaine than to lidocaine, which can be used in most patients allergic to procaine. Anaphylactic reactions to these drugs may occur in patients who are unaware of previous allergic episodes. The operator should have on hand an emergency kit for the treatment of such reactions. This kit must contain epinephrine, hydrocortisone for intravenous use, and an airway. If a cardiac standstill occurs during an anaphylactic reaction, resuscitation measures have to be instituted immediately.

For local anesthesia, about 3 ml of a 2% lidocaine solution are drawn through a 20 gauge needle into a 5 ml syringe provided with a Luer-

Lok. A 25 gauge needle is then substituted, and an intradermal injection producing a 5 mm papule is performed. The operator then changes to a 20 gauge needle, which is placed through the papule onto the periosteum. With the needle on the periosteum, about 1.0 ml of lidocaine is injected. The needle is withdrawn and a bone marrow needle is pushed through the skin down to the periosteum. We routinely use the 1 inch, gauge 16 or 18 Osgood needle (Becton, Dickinson & Co., Rutherford, N.J.). In practice, any bone marrow needle can be used. Preferably it should have a stylet fixed by a Luer-Lok or similar device. An inch-long needle is adequate for most patients, except those with a thick layer of subcutaneous fat tissue; the outer portion of the Vim-Silverman needle may be used in these cases. A gauge 16 or 18 needle can be easily introduced through the skin without incision and yields excellent particles. The needle and stylet are pushed into the bone with a rotary, alternating clockwise and counterclockwise motion, the needle being directed toward the anterior superior iliac spine. When the needle is firmly placed, the stylet is withdrawn and a 20 ml disposable plastic syringe is attached. Plastic syringes produce more suction than glass syringes because of the tighter fit of the plunger. The plunger of the syringe is then pulled back vigorously and about 10 ml of marrow mixed with blood are aspirated. The patient should be warned that he will experience an unpleasant sensation or some pain when the plunger of the syringe is pulled back. This unpleasant feeling is much stronger when marrow is aspirated from the sternum.

Almost all the aspirated marrow is immediately discharged into a 4 ounce, wide-mouthed, screw-cap jar (H. H. Thomas Co., Philadelphia, Pa., catalogue no. 6284-F) containing approximately 2 ounces of a neutral, buffered, 10% formalin solution [12]. About 0.2 ml of marrow retained in the syringe is then discharged onto the raised end of a slide elevated 1 cm by resting it on the screw cap of the specimen bottle, while the other end of the slide rests on another slide (Fig. 1-2). On the inclined slide the peripheral blood runs down, leaving behind bone marrow particles on the upper half of the slide. These are picked up with the short edge of a slide and smeared across another slide, which is held between the index finger and thumb while it rests securely on the middle finger (Fig. 1-3). The only pressure applied to the smeared-out particle should be the weight of the slide.

If desired, imprints of bone marrow particles or coverslip smears can be prepared at this point. Those who prefer smears of dilute marrow to crushed particle smears can deposit one drop of the remaining aspirated marrow on slides and prepare smears in the usual way. We prefer crushed particle smears because the hematopoietic cells are more concentrated and mast cells can be evaluated in the thick areas. The prepared slides are air dried and stained with a mixture of Harleco's Wright and Giemsa stains (Harleco, Philadelphia, Pa.) (see Appendix, 6). The optimum fixing and staining times vary somewhat from batch to batch; they should be determined for each new batch of stain. The staining and fixation times are approximately twice as long for bone marrows as for

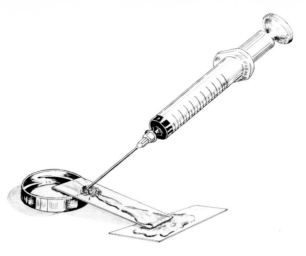

Figure 1-2
Slanted slide rests on the screw cap of the specimen bottle and on another slide. After most of the aspirated bone marrow has been ejected into a jar containing formalin, the remaining marrow is discharged onto the elevated part of the slanted slide. Bone marrow particles are seen on upper half of slide after the peripheral blood has run down onto the other slide.

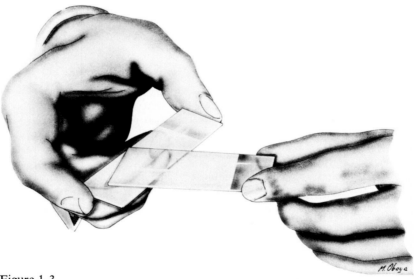

Figure 1-3
Bone marrow particles are picked up with the short edge of a slide and are smeared across another slide held between the index finger and thumb and resting securely on the middle finger.

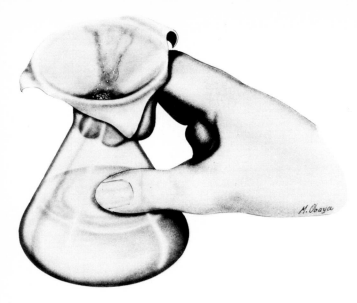

Figure 1-4
The contents of the specimen bottle are poured into a funnel containing a filter paper prepared from a Templefiber Tissue Filter Bag. The specimen jar is rinsed with formalin, which is also poured through the filter. The peripheral blood passes through, while the particles are left behind.

peripheral blood smears. All smears are coverslipped for protection and for viewing with medium and high dry magnifications.

If recent peripheral blood smears are not available, they should be obtained at this time.

The bottle containing the bone marrow particles is taken to the histopathology laboratory, where the entire specimen is poured through a small funnel containing a filter prepared from the rectangular, 4½ × 3 inch paper obtained by removing the seams of a disposable Templefiber tissue bag (Templefiber Tissue Filter Bags, Temple T. Co., Philadelphia, Pa.). The bottle is rinsed with formalin, which is then also poured through the funnel (Fig. 1-4). Because of the porosity of the filter paper, the red cells and some of the polymorphonuclear leukocytes pass through while the particles are left behind. The material caught in the filter paper is washed several times with formalin squeezed from a plastic wash bottle. The particles are washed into a clump, after which the filter paper is folded and enclosed in a tissue capsule and processed in the Autotechnicon. We routinely cut 10 sections 5 to 6 μ thick. The fourth and seventh sections, as well as one of the smears, are stained with Gomori's method for iron (see Appendix, 2) [13] and the remaining sections with hematoxylin and eosin. Special stains such as Gordon-Sweets' method or the PAS reaction (see Appendix, 3, 7) or the van Gieson stain are performed when necessary. To reiterate, the principle of our technic is to concentrate the bone marrow particles by separating them from the peripheral blood [14]. This is accomplished by ejecting the aspirate, before it clots, into a formaldehyde solution. Other fixatives, such as Zenker's, Maximow's, Bouin's, and Schaudinn's, lake the red cells and make it impossible to wash them through the Templefiber bag, and thus yield a lesser concentration of particles; their use, however, results in better cytologic detail. Nonetheless, in general their disadvantages outweigh their advantages. Absolute alcohol must be used as the fixative when cystinosis is suspected. Smears are prepared from particles sticking to the slanted slide after the peripheral blood has run down.

We aspirate more marrow (about 10 ml) than is usually recommended (0.5–1 ml). It is true that the additional aspirate contains fewer particles than the initial 0.5 ml. However, because we concentrate the particles by filtration, we end up with more particles by aspirating additional bone marrow even though it is more dilute.

Aspirated particles processed in the manner described yield a better histologic preparation than so-called clot sections of bone marrow. In the latter, the histologic sections contain scanty particles separated by erythrocytes and fibrin clots. Our method yields many bone marrow particles lying side by side without intervening erythrocytes or fibrin clots (Fig. 1-5).

When the slide tray is submitted to the hematopathologist for interpretation it contains: 10 slides with sections of bone marrow particles, 8 stained with hematoxylin and eosin and 2 stained for iron; 3 smears of crushed particles, 1 stained for iron and 2 stained with a Wright-Giemsa mixture; and a peripheral blood smear. All the smears are coverslipped. An iron control is submitted with each batch of specimens. The tissue slip submitted with the bone marrow contains significant information about the history, physical examination, and other pertinent laboratory data. A copy of the complete blood count (CBC) report is attached.

Needle Biopsy of Bone Marrow and Bone

A bone marrow and bone biopsy are indicated either when the needle aspiration of the bone marrow results in a dry tap, that is, no bone marrow particles can be aspirated, or when there is a specific indication to study bone histology. The former occurs in myelofibrosis, the latter when bone disorders such as Paget's disease or hyperparathyroidism are suspected.

We find that a nonincisional needle biopsy, done as easily as an aspiration, yields excellent results. A number of different needles have been recommended: Turkel (V. Mueller & Co., Atlanta, Ga.) [15], Westerman-Jensen (Becton, Dickinson & Co., Rutherford, N.J.) [6], Gardner (special product, Becton, Dickinson & Co.), Vim-Silverman (Becton, Dickinson & Co.) [4], and others.

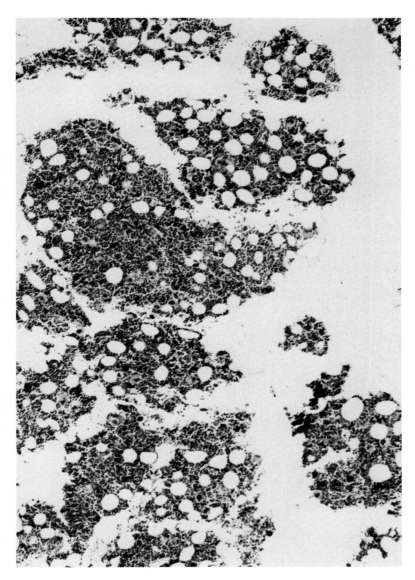

Figure 1-5
Appearance of concentrated bone marrow particles in histologic sections of aspirated marrow. Note absence of admixed blood. (H&E, ×79.)

For a number of years we have used the same Osgood needle that we use for aspiration of the bone marrow. The technic is identical with that described for bone marrow aspiration. After the stylet is withdrawn, the needle is advanced into the bone in the direction of the anterior superior iliac spine in the usual manner. When it has penetrated deep enough, the needle is rotated clockwise and counterclockwise through a few complete turns in an attempt to cut the distal attachment of the tissue cylinder, which is inside the lumen of the needle. The needle is then withdrawn and the tissue within the lumen of the needle is pushed out by reintroducing the stylet. The tissue fragment is dropped directly into a specimen jar containing a neutral, buffered, 10% formalin solution. The specimen is decalcified and processed through the Autotechnicon. Examples of such biopsies are shown in Figures 1-6 to 1-8. Dr. Carlos Dominguez discovered this technic by serendipity during his residency in our department. He withdrew the stylet too early while performing a bone marrow aspiration and obtained a dry tap. The needle was clogged by what proved to be a very acceptable bone and marrow specimen.

In recent years we have utilized the regular adult 11 gauge Jamshidi needle, which yields very good biopsy specimens [11]. It is used the same way as described for the Osgood needle, except that the specimen is pushed out of the needle by introducing a probe through the distal cutting end.

Burkhardt [3] has described an incisional bone and marrow biopsy method using a plastic embedding medium and a special microtome capable of cutting undecalcified bone. Beautiful preparations are obtained. This method represents a surgical biopsy; the skin incision has to be sutured or clipped and the patient kept off work for 3 days. In our experience, surgical bone marrow biopsy is rarely, if ever, required in hematologic cases. Needle biopsies of bone and bone marrow have been studied extensively by Duhamel [5].

Histologic sections of aspirated bone marrow particles are in many ways superior to those prepared from specimens obtained by biopsy. The latter require decalcification and often show crushing artifacts that result in decreased cytologic detail. The Giemsa stain is difficult and the Leder stain impossible to perform on decalcified tissue (see Appendix). More marrow is obtained by our technic than by biopsy with a 14 gauge Franklin-Silverman needle or an 11 gauge Jamshidi needle, as was shown by Ioannides and Rywlin [10] by obtaining aspirated marrow from one posterior superior iliac spine and a biopsy from the opposite side in 30 cadavers. Weight and a point-counting technic were utilized to evaluate the amount of marrow obtained. Biopsy by the Jamshidi needle was superior to that using the Franklin-Silverman needle [10].

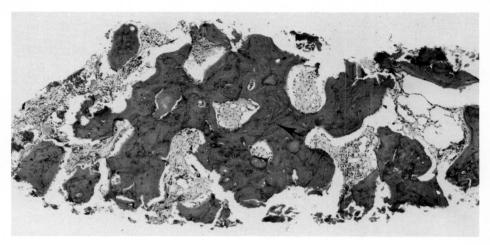

Figure 1-6
Example of bone marrow biopsy obtained with a 16 gauge Osgood needle, the same needle that is used for aspiration of bone marrow, showing Paget's disease. Note fibrosis of marrow and increased number of cementing lines (*arrow*), which are responsible for mosaic appearance of bone. (H&E, ×45.)

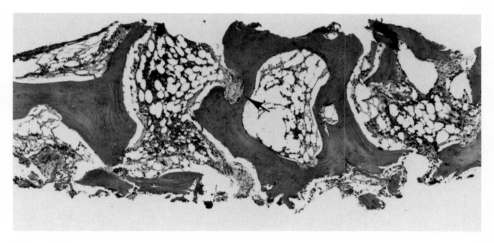

Figure 1-7
Bone marrow biopsy obtained with Osgood needle, showing osteitis fibrosa. Note tonguelike fibrous resorption of bone (*arrow*). (H&E, ×45.)

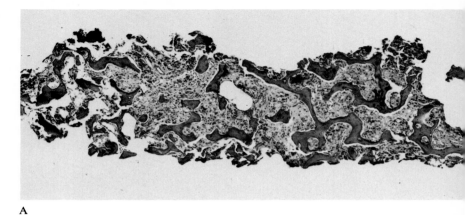

A

B

Figure 1-8
Osgood needle biopsies: (A) Metastatic carcinoma. Marrow is devoid of fat
cells and is infiltrated by carcinoma cells (see B). (H&E, ×45.) (B) Higher
power of A, showing details of undifferentiated carcinoma. (H&E, ×396.)

References

1. Arinkin, M. I. Die intravitale Untersuchungsmethodik des Knochenmarks. *Folia Haematol.* 38:233, 1929.
2. Bakir, F. Fatal sternal puncture: Report of a case. *Dis. Chest* 44:435, 1963.
3. Burkhardt, R. *Farbatlas der klinischen Histopathologie von Knochenmark und Knochen.* Berlin, Heidelberg, New York: Springer, 1970.
4. Conrad, M. E., Jr., and Crosby, W. H. Bone marrow biopsy: Modification of the Vim-Silverman needle. *J. Lab. Clin. Med.* 57:642, 1961.
5. Duhamel, G. *Histopathologie clinique de la moëlle osseuse.* Paris: Masson, 1974.
6. Ellis, L. D., Jensen, W. N., and Westerman, M. F. Needle biopsy of bone and marrow: An experience with 1,445 biopsies. *Arch. Intern. Med.* 114:213, 1964.
7. Fine, N. L., Reich, E. J., and Weinsaft, P. Growth of sternal tumor mass following bone marrow aspiration. *N.Y. State J. Med.* 67:2866, 1967.
8. Garnier, H., Reynier, J., and Dimopoulos, F. A propos des accidents de la ponction sternale. *Ann. Chir.* 18:308, 1964.
9. Gildenhorn, L. H., Gildenhorn, B. V., and Amromin, G. Marrow embolism and intraosseous contrast radiography. *J.A.M.A.* 173:758, 1960.
10. Ioannides, K., and Rywlin, A. M. A comparative study of histologic sections of bone marrow obtained by aspiration and by needle biopsy (abstract). *Am. J. Clin. Pathol.* 65:267, 1976.
11. Jamshidi, K., and Swaim, W. R. Bone marrow biopsy with unaltered architecture: A new biopsy device. *J. Lab. Clin. Med.* 77:335, 1971.
12. Lillie, R. D. *Histopathologic Technic and Practical Histochemistry* (3rd ed.). New York: Blakiston Div., McGraw-Hill, 1965. P. 38.
13. Luna, L. E. *Manual of Histologic Staining Methods of the Armed Forces Institute of Pathology* (3rd ed.). New York: McGraw-Hill, 1968. P. 179.
14. Rywlin, A. M., Marvan, P., and Robinson, M. J. A simple technic for the preparation of bone marrow smears and sections. *Am. J. Clin. Pathol.* 53:389, 1970.
15. Turkel, H., and Bethell, F. H. Biopsy of bone marrow performed by a new and simple instrument. *J. Lab. Clin. Med.* 28:1246, 1943.
16. Wintrobe, M. M. *Clinical Hematology* (6th ed.). Philadelphia: Lea & Febiger, 1967. P. 36.
17. Yoell, J. H. Bone marrow embolism to lung following sternal puncture. *Arch. Pathol.* 67:373, 1959.

2 The Bone Marrow Report

The bone marrow report is made up of three parts: description, diagnosis, and comment.

Description

The description summarizes in an orderly fashion morphologic observations made on the peripheral blood smear and on the bone marrow sections and smears. In the training of our residents, we insist that a definite order be followed in the examination of blood smears and bone marrow preparations, to avoid being mesmerized by a striking abnormality of one cell series and overlooking associated pathologic findings in other cells. We always examine the peripheral blood and the bone marrow preparation first with a medium power objective and then with the high dry lens. In order to do this, the peripheral blood and bone marrow smears must be coverslipped unless special objectives are available. The oil-immersion magnification is used only for certain nuclear or cytologic details; it is not used routinely for the examination of every case. Virtually all diagnoses can be made with the high dry objective.

Examination of the peripheral smear consists of a systematic study of the platelets and red and white blood cells. Smears prepared from blood obtained by fingertip puncture are superior to those made from anticoagulated blood. With some experience it becomes easy to decide whether the number of platelets is normal, increased, or decreased. Beginners might be guided by the following principle [1]: If there are several platelets in almost every oil-immersion field with occasional clumps, platelets are regarded as being numerically adequate; less than one platelet per oil-immersion field is considered a decrease and more than 25 platelets per oil-immersion field an increase in number. The morphology of the platelets is also studied.

After the platelets, the morphology of the red cells is examined. A well-prepared peripheral smear has a thick area at one end, where the drop of blood was applied, and a thin, feathery edge at the other end of the slide. Red cell morphology should be studied in the portion of the smear close to the feathery edge where the red cells are evenly spaced and overlap occasionally. The white cells are studied with respect to their numbers and morphology. The total leukocyte count can be estimated from the differential smear by using Dorsey's table (Table 2-1) [1]. With some experience, it becomes easy to decide from the peripheral smear whether the leukocyte count is normal, increased, or decreased.

The examination of the peripheral smear helps greatly in interpreting the bone marrow findings. In addition, for the physician supervising a hematology laboratory, examination of the peripheral smear is an excel-

Table 2-1. Estimation of Total Leukocyte Count from the Differential Smear [1]

Average No. Leukocytes (per high-power field)	Total Leukocyte Count (per mm³)
2–4	4,000–7,000
4–6	7,000–10,000
6–10	10,000–13,000
10–20	13,000–18,000

Source: Reprinted with permission from D. B. Dorsey, Quality control in hematology. *American Journal of Clinical Pathology* 40:457, 1963.

lent means of quality control. By comparing his findings with those reported by the technologist on the complete blood count (CBC) report, the physician gets a good idea of the competence of his technologists.

The bone marrow description is a result of the study of sections and smears. We do not describe the sections and smears separately. In describing the bone marrow, we follow this order:

1. Cellularity
2. Megakaryocytes
3. Red cells
4. Hemosiderin content
5. E:G ratio (nucleated red cells:granulocytes; also called M:E [myeloid:erythroid] ratio)
6. Granulocytes
7. Eosinophils
8. Plasma cells
9. Mast cells
10. Lymphocytes
11. Stromal reactions, including serous atrophy of fat, vascular lesions, inflammatory reactions, necrosis, granulomas, increase in reticulin framework, and fibrosis
12. Foreign cells and parasites

These items are discussed in some detail in subsequent chapters.

A normal bone marrow report reads as follows:

The peripheral blood smear shows no abnormalities of platelets or red or white cells.

The bone marrow particles are normocellular. Megakaryocytes are normal in number and morphology. The red cell series is normoblastic. Hemosiderin granules are present. The E:G ratio is within normal limits. The granulocytic series shows normal maturation. Eosinophils and plasma and mast cells are unremarkable. There are no lymphoid nodules. No vascular lesions, granulomas, foreign cells, or parasites are seen.

Diagnosis

Following the description of the bone marrow, we make a diagnosis. The diagnosis is a morphologic one, i.e., it is based solely on the observations that we have made on the peripheral blood smear and the bone marrow preparations. Thus, if we saw megaloblastic erythropoiesis, giant metamyelocytes, and hypersegmented polymorphonuclear leukocytes, these findings would be recorded under the diagnoses. For example:

Diagnoses:
  Megaloblastic erythropoiesis
  Giant metamyelocytes
  Hypersegmented polymorphonuclear leukocytes

For coding purposes, it is convenient to record these findings under separate headings.

Our diagnosis is a summary of the description and is simply an enumeration of the abnormalities observed in the peripheral blood and bone marrow.

Comment

Following the diagnosis, we write a brief comment, if indicated. In the above example of a megaloblastic erythropoiesis, the comment might read as follows:

Comment: The above findings are consistent with the clinical diagnosis of pernicious anemia. A Schilling test and a search for antibodies for intrinsic factor should be performed to confirm the diagnosis. Vitamin B_{12} and folic acid levels would also be helpful.

The purpose of the comment is to correlate the morphologic observations with clinical and laboratory findings. Additional clinical and laboratory data may be necessary to understand the morphologic observations. Thus, for example, finding metastatic carcinoma cells suggestive of a prostatic primary will prompt a request for an acid and alkaline phosphatase determination.

Reference

1. Dorsey, D. B.   Quality control in hematology. *Am. J. Clin. Pathol.* 40:457, 1963.

3 Bone Marrow Cellularity

Yellow and Red Marrow

There are two types of bone marrow which can be clearly distinguished macroscopically: yellow marrow and red marrow. Yellow marrow is made up of mature fat cells (adipocytes). Red marrow consists of varying mixtures of adipocytes and hematopoietic cells, the latter including cells of the megakaryocytic, erythrocytic, and granulocytic series with an admixture of lymphocytes and plasma, reticulum, and mast cells. The red color of the bone marrow is determined by cells of the erythrocytic series as well as by the amount of blood in the sinusoids [1].

In the newborn, the entire bone marrow is red and contains no fat cells [1]. After birth, red marrow is gradually replaced by yellow marrow. The replacement starts in the distal segments of the extremities and proceeds centripetally until it reaches the proximal segments of the humerus and femur. In the normal adult, red marrow is found in the skull, clavicles, scapulae, sternum, ribs, spine, pelvis, and proximal segments of the humerus and femur. A few small islands of red marrow can be found elsewhere in the long bones [1]. This distribution of red marrow has been confirmed by scintiphotographs of the positron-emitting isotope ^{52}Fe [6].

General Concepts

The concept of bone marrow cellularity is based on the relative amounts of hematopoietic and fat cells in bone marrow particles (Figs. 3-1 to 3-3). The hematopoietic marrow is commonly referred to as "cellular" marrow. This term, though not quite correct because the fatty marrow is also made up of cells, is generally accepted. The data as to what constitutes normal bone marrow cellularity are scanty. In the newborn and during the first years of life, there are no adipocytes in the vertebral bone marrow [5]. In the normal adult, about one-third of the hematopoietic bone marrow is fatty [5]. Additional quantitative studies are needed to determine normal bone marrow cellularity, taking into consideration such factors as site of aspiration, nutritional status, and age of the patient. Such studies may be performed using morphometric technics, as described by Weibel and Elias [7]. Hartsock et al. [4] determined the cellularity of bone marrow from the anterior iliac crest by a point-counting method. They found a 79 percent cellularity during the first decade of life; it diminished to about 50 percent at the age of 30 years and remained relatively constant until age 70 years. During the eighth decade, an appreciable decline in the amount of hematopoietic tissue occurred [4].

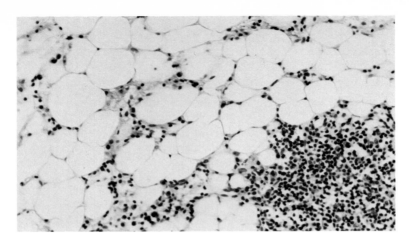

Figure 3-1
Hypocellular marrow. Sparsity of hematopoietic elements and predominance of fat cells. Note lymphoid nodule in lower right corner. Seventy-year-old woman with Hgb 9.9 gm/100 ml, WBC 1,350/mm³, and platelets 2,000/mm³. (H&E, ×176.)

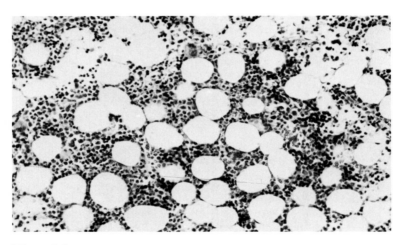

Figure 3-2
Normocellular marrow. Ninety-one-year-old man with bronchogenic carcinoma. Note that fat cells occupy close to 50 percent of the surface area of the bone marrow particle. (H&E, ×176.)

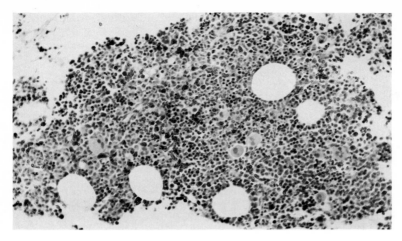

Figure 3-3
Hypercellular marrow. Sixty-five-year-old woman with polycythemia vera. Note the sparsity of fat cells and the obvious hyperplasia of the megakaryocytic series. (H&E, ×176.)

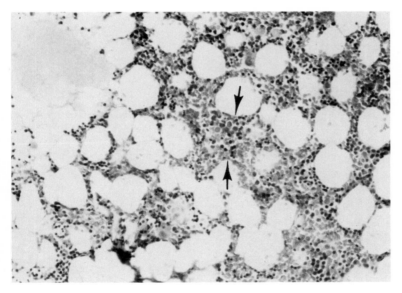

Figure 3-4
Hypocellular marrow without increase in the number of fat cells. Spaces separating fat cells are occupied predominantly by red blood cells. Hematopoietic cells are markedly decreased (*between arrows*). (H&E, ×160.)

21

In addition to the number of fat cells per unit area, bone marrow cellularity also depends on how tightly the hematopoietic cells are packed. It is possible to have a hypocellular marrow because of a decrease of hematopoietic elements without an increase in fat cells. The hematopoietic cells may be replaced by red blood cells, as seen in marrow hemorrhages, or by fibrin as in fibrinous myelitis (Fig. 3-4). Hypercellular marrows without a decrease in the number of fat cells are seen in some chronic lymphocytic leukemias in which normal hematopoietic cells are replaced by tightly packed lymphocytes (see Chap. 9).

Normal Cellularity

In our experience, particles aspirated from the posterior superior iliac spine may vary in cellularity from 25 to 75 percent in the presence of normal peripheral blood findings. In addition, there is considerable variability in the cellularity of different particles in the same bone marrow aspirate (Figs. 3-5, 3-6). Occasionally, a particle composed entirely of fat cells may be associated with more highly cellular particles, or markedly hypercellular particles may be associated with normocellular or hypocellular particles in the same aspirate. Cellularity also varies at different sites of aspiration. Hartsock et al. [4] concluded that the amount of hematopoietic tissue of the anterior iliac crest is greater than that of the rib and less than that of the sternum. Because of these

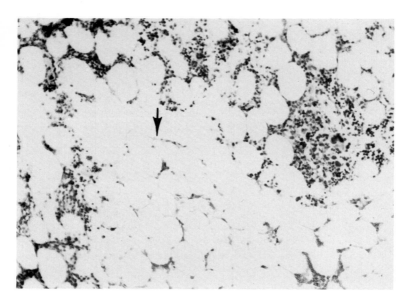

Figure 3-5
Hypocellular particle (*arrow*) adjacent to normocellular marrow in the same bone marrow aspirate. (H&E, ×176.)

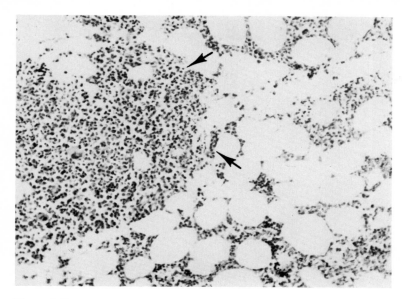

Figure 3-6
Hypercellular particle (*arrows*) adjacent to normocellular marrow in the same bone marrow aspirate. (H&E, ×176.)

considerations, it must be realized that there are limitations in drawing conclusions about such a large organ as the bone marrow on the basis of the relatively small samples obtained by aspiration or biopsy technics.

It is both easier and much more accurate to estimate cellularity from histologic sections than from smears. Histologic sections are also superior to bone marrow hematocrit determinations in the estimation of cellularity, because dilution problems are eliminated. With a simple morphometric device such as the point-counting system of Chaulkley [2], statistically significant results can be obtained.

Though normal cellularity is difficult to define in exact terms because of the absence of adequate data, marked deviations from the normal are easily appreciated from the study of histologic material. Disturbances in cellularity may result in hypocellular (hypoplastic) or hypercellular (hyperplastic) marrows (see Figs. 3-1 to 3-3).

Hypocellular Marrow

Figure 3-1 represents a hypocellular marrow. The major part of the volume of each bone marrow particle is represented by normal fat cells. The cellular components of hypoplastic marrows must be studied carefully, because the different cell series may not be affected to the same degree. It is important to know that acute leukemia may present with a hypocellular marrow. The finding of increased numbers of blasts, associated with abnormal cellular maturation, will help in establishing the

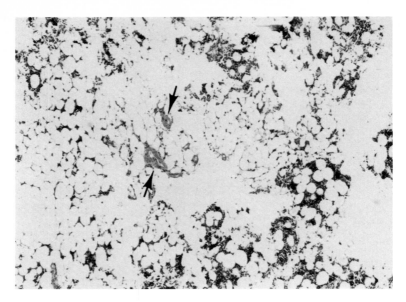

Figure 3-7
Focus of hypocellular marrow centered by blood vessels (*arrows*). (H&E, ×50.)

diagnosis. Cytologically normal lymphoid nodules may be present in increased numbers in hypocellular marrows, representing an absolute increase, rather than a relative prominence, because of atrophy of other elements. Plasma, mast, and reticulum cells are often quite prominent in hypocellular marrows. This probably represents a relative as well as an absolute increase. Conditions which may give rise to hypocellular marrows are listed below. Occasionally foci of hypocellular marrow are centered around blood vessels; the significance of this finding is not clear (Fig. 3-7).

Hypocellular (Hypoplastic) Bone Marrow

Physiologic state (e.g.: site of aspiration, old age)
Radiation therapy
Chemotherapy
Drugs
Toxins
Infectious hepatitis [3]
Some refractory anemias
Some leukemias
Paroxysmal nocturnal hemoglobinuria
Fanconi's syndrome (familial constitutional panmyelocytopathy)
Miliary tuberculosis
Hypoplasia of single cell series (discussed in subsequent chapters)

Hypercellular Marrow

Hypercellular or hyperplastic marrows may be seen under different circumstances (see following list).

Hypercellular (Hyperplastic) Bone Marrow

Physiologic state (e.g.: newborn)
Polycythemia vera
Erythroleukemia
Some refractory anemias
Pernicious anemia
Severe hemolytic anemia
Megakaryocytic myelosis
Leukemias
Leukemoid reactions
Hypersplenism
Tuberculosis
Hyperplasia of single cell series (discussed in subsequent chapters)

A careful and systematic study of the bone marrow will usually lead to a diagnosis. Minor degrees of hypercellularity may be difficult to recognize. It is also important to decide whether all cell series or only one particular cell series is hyperplastic. These considerations are discussed in more detail in subsequent chapters.

Hypercellular marrows may show either a normal distribution of cells with a predominance of mature forms or a predominance of immature cells. The predominance of immature cells seems to be due to a compensatory hyperplasia of the proliferating (dividing) compartment of a cell series rather than to a "maturation arrest," i.e., an interference with maturation of cells in the "differentiating" (maturation) compartment of a cell series.

References

1. Askanazy, M.   Knochenmark. In F. Henke and O. Lubarsch (Eds.), *Handbuch der speziellen pathologischen Anatomie und Histologie*. Berlin: Springer, 1927. Vol. 1, pt. 2, pp. 775–779.
2. Chaulkley, H. W.   Method for the quantitative morphologic analysis of tissues. *J. Natl. Cancer Inst.* 4:47, 1943.
3. Editorial.   Infectious hepatitis and aplastic anemia. *Lancet* 1:844, 1971.
4. Hartsock, R. J., Smith, E. B., and Petty, C. S.   Normal variations with aging of the amount of hematopoietic tissue in bone marrow from the anterior iliac crest. *Am. J. Clin. Pathol.* 43:326, 1965.
5. Lennert, K.   Zur Praxis der pathologisch-anatomischen Knochenmarksuntersuchung. *Frankf. Z. Pathol.* 63:267, 1952.
6. Van Dyke, D., and Anger, H. O.   Patterns of marrow hypertrophy and atrophy in man. *J. Nucl. Med.* 6:109, 1965.
7. Weibel, E. R., and Elias, H.   *Quantitative Methods in Morphology*. Berlin: Springer, 1967.

4 Megakaryocytes

Morphology

The megakaryocyte can be easily identified in histologic sections of bone marrow particles. The largest cell present, it can be spotted under low power. It appears as a multinucleated cell, but closer inspection reveals that the nucleus is multilobed and convoluted (Fig. 4-1). The nucleus is rich in chromatin, and nucleoli cannot be clearly distinguished. The cytoplasm is eosinophilic and the nuclear-cytoplasmic ratio varies. The cytoplasm is PAS positive before and after treatment with diastase. Large, intensely PAS positive cytoplasmic granules and ingested red blood cells, or polymorphonuclear leukocytes, are seen occasionally (Figs. 4-2, 4-3). Frequently, naked megakaryocytic nuclei are encountered, showing varying degrees of pyknosis (Fig. 4-4). The megakaryocyte precursors, megakaryoblasts and promegakaryocytes, cannot be recognized with certainty in bone marrow sections.

Platelets appear in histologic sections as a granular, eosinophilic material that should not be confused with precipitated fibrin. Fibrin is also eosinophilic, but it shows a threadlike arrangement. Furthermore, fibrin is gram positive and stains with phosphotungstic acid–hematoxylin. When there is increased platelet production, sheets of platelets can be seen assuming peculiar shapes. These sheets of platelets may be surrounded by one or two rows of polymorphonuclear leukocytes (Figs. 4-5, 7-4). The cause of this attraction of polymorphonuclear leukocytes by platelets is unknown.

In sections of bone marrow particles it is impossible to confuse megakaryocytes with other giant cells. Reed-Sternberg cells have prominent eosinophilic nucleoli surrounded by a clear halo (Fig. 4-6). Osteoclasts have many discrete nuclei and a more basophilic cytoplasm (Fig. 4-7). Langhans-type giant cells show a horseshoelike arrangement of nuclei (Fig. 4-8). Foreign-body giant cells display central concentration of nuclei and either surround or contain foreign bodies (Figs. 4-9 to 4-11). Touton giant cells show a peripheral vacuolization of the cytoplasm (Fig. 4-12). Furthermore, the location of giant cells aids in their identification. Megakaryocytes occur among other normal marrow elements; Reed-Sternberg cells are seen in association with other cells suggestive of Hodgkin's disease (see Chap. 9). Osteoclasts lie in Howship's lacunae (see Fig. 4-7), tumor giant cells are accompanied by other neoplastic cells, and Langhans' cells are associated with granulomas (see Chap. 11).

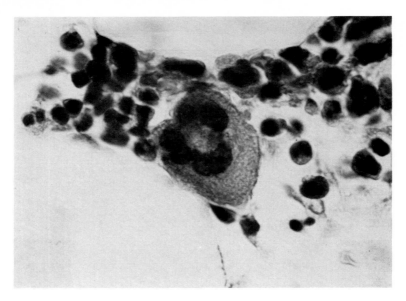

Figure 4-1
Normal megakaryocyte. Note multilobed nucleus. (H&E, ×1146.)

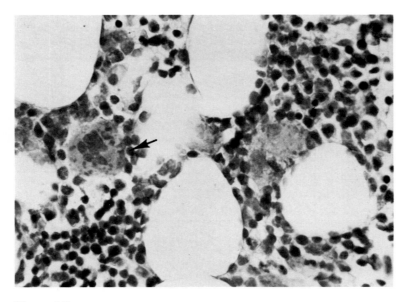

Figure 4-2
PAS-positive granules in cytoplasm of megakaryocyte (*arrow*). (PAS, ×494.)

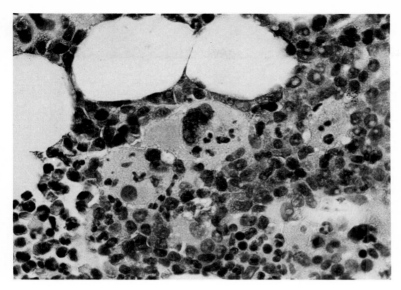

Figure 4-3
Megakaryocytes with ingested polymorphonuclear leukocytes. (H&E, ×494.)

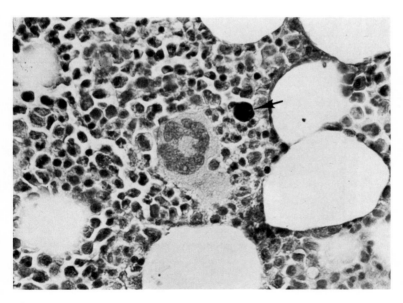

Figure 4-4
Pyknotic megakaryocyte (*arrow*) adjacent to normal megakaryocyte. (H&E, ×454.)

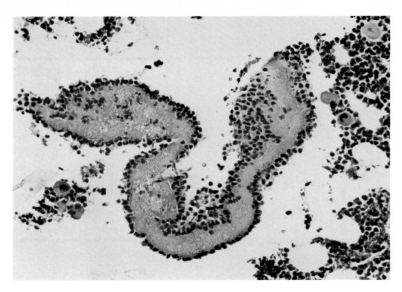

Figure 4-5
Serpentine configuration of clumped platelets surrounded by polymorphonuclear leukocytes (see also Fig. 7-4). (H&E, ×189.)

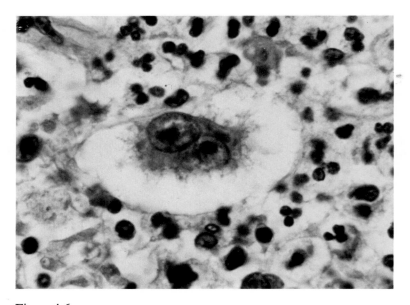

Figure 4-6
Reed-Sternberg cell. Note prominent nucleoli. The clear cytoplasmic area is characteristic of the lacunar type of Reed-Sternberg cell seen in the nodular sclerosis variant of Hodgkin's disease. (H&E, ×1146.)

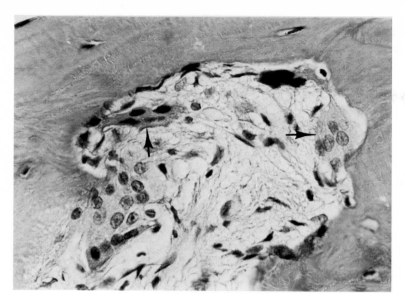

Figure 4-7
Osteoclasts (*arrows*). Right osteoclast lies in Howship's lacuna. (H&E, ×524.)

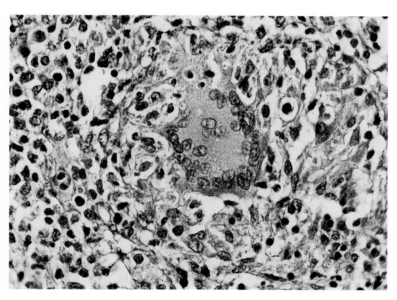

Figure 4-8
Langhans' giant cell in tuberculous granuloma. (H&E, ×424.)

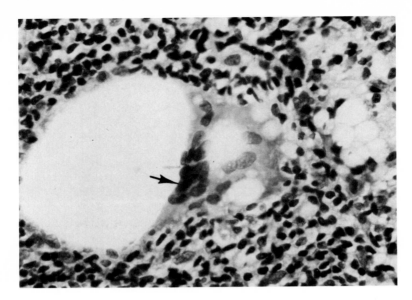

Figure 4-9
Foreign-body-type multinucleated cell (*arrow*) in lipid granuloma. Empty spaces represent fat dissolved by embedding process. (H&E, ×524.)

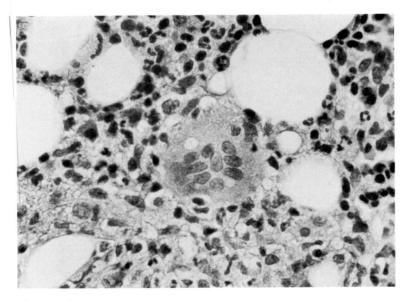

Figure 4-10
Foreign body giant cell associated with suppurative granuloma of unknown etiology. (H&E, ×524.)

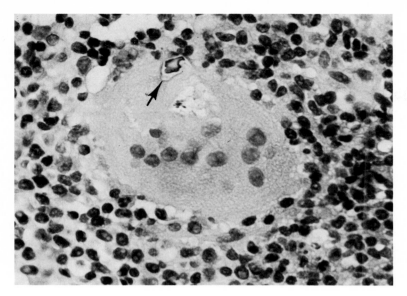

Figure 4-11
Foreign body giant cell with crystalline inclusion (*arrow*). (H&E, ×588.)

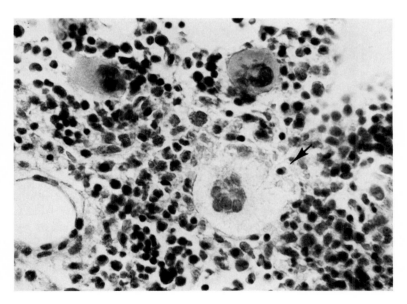

Figure 4-12
Touton giant cell (*arrow*) in a 20-year-old diabetic woman with type IV hyperlipoproteinemia. Note characteristic vacuolated periphery. (H&E, ×459.)

33

Numerical Considerations

No exact information is available as to the normal number of megakaryocytes per unit area of hematopoietic marrow; striking deviations from normal, such as complete absence or marked increase of megakaryocytes, are easily appreciated. Minor deviations have to be evaluated carefully, particularly because there is considerable variation in numbers of megakaryocytes from particle to particle.

Conditions in which megakaryocytes are numerically altered are listed below.

Megakaryocytes

Increased	Decreased
Polycythemia vera	Congenital aplasia
Chronic granulocytic leukemia	Acute leukemias
Megakaryocytic myelosis	Agnogenic myeloid metaplasia
Essential thrombocythemia	Neoplasias
Some refractory anemias	Radiation
Metastatic carcinoma	Toxins
Hodgkin's disease	Alcoholism
Hemorrhage	Drugs
Hemolysis	Infections
After splenectomy	Pernicious anemia
Hypersplenism	Aplastic anemia
Infections	
Agranulocytosis	
Asphyxia	
Carcinoid syndrome (?)	
Idiopathic thrombocytopenic purpura	
Thrombotic thrombocytopenic purpura	
Sarcoidosis	

Decreased megakaryocytes are always associated with thrombocytopenia. Increased megakaryocytes may be seen with normal, decreased, or increased numbers of platelets in the peripheral blood. In acute leukemia the megakaryocytes, as a rule, are markedly decreased; occasionally, they are highly atypical and are increased in number (Fig. 4-13). The differential diagnosis between acute leukemia and a "blast crisis" of chronic granulocytic leukemia has to be considered in such instances. In a blast crisis of chronic granulocytic leukemia, megakaryocytes are present in larger numbers than in acute leukemia. In pernicious anemia or other vitamin B_{12} or folic acid deficiencies, the bone marrow may show decreased megakaryocytes with hypersegmented forms (Fig. 4-14).

Most of the drugs that can cause thrombocytopenia do so by destroying megakaryocytes. A few drugs (quinidine, chlorothiazide) are responsible for destruction of platelets [1].

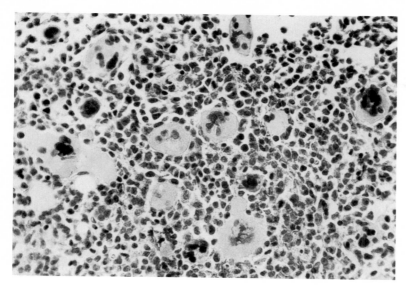

Figure 4-13
Numerically increased and atypical megakaryocytes in acute blastic leukemia.
(H&E, ×308).

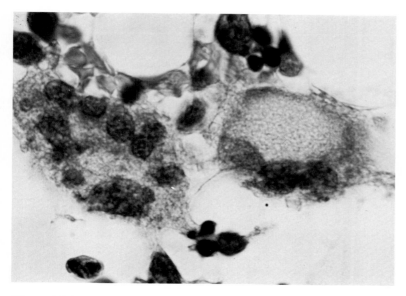

Figure 4-14
Hypersegmented megakaryocyte in pernicious anemia. (H&E, ×1411.)

In chronic granulocytic leukemia there is marked megakaryocytic hyperplasia. The megakaryocytes appear normal or may actually be somewhat smaller than normal [3, 5]. In polycythemia vera, the megakaryocytes are increased in number and are surrounded by reticulin fibers (Figs. 4-15, 4-16). Furthermore, the megakaryocytes often appear larger than normal [3, 5]. Also, in contrast to chronic granulocytic leukemia, there is a striking erythroblastic hyperplasia and the hemosiderin stores are depleted.

In agnogenic myeloid metaplasia, megakaryocytes are increased in number and are surrounded by reticulin or collagen fibers (Fig. 4-17). In idiopathic thrombocythemia (essential thrombocythemia) there is marked hyperplasia of megakaryocytes with preservation of fat cells (Fig. 4-18). Fat cells are usually markedly decreased or absent in polycythemia vera and in chronic granulocytic leukemia (see Fig. 4-15). Essential thrombocythemia runs a chronic course with a sustained and pronounced thrombocytosis.

Acute megakaryocytic myelosis (acute megakaryocytic leukemia) is a rapidly progressive disease characterized by the proliferation of atypical, neoplastic-appearing megakaryocytes [6, 7] (Fig. 4-19). It may be associated with thrombocytosis or thrombocytopenia. Red cell and granulocytic precursors may be markedly atypical [2]. A variant of this entity has been described by Guichard et al. [4] as "aleukemic decalci-

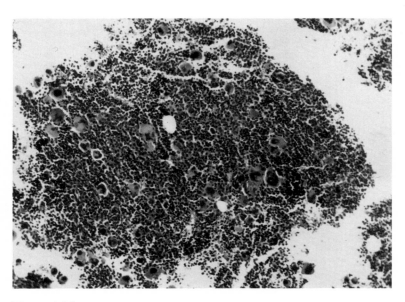

Figure 4-15
Increased megakaryocytes in a hypercellular marrow in polycythemia vera. (H&E, ×114.)

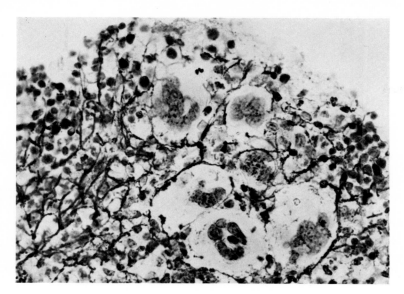

Figure 4-16
Polycythemia vera. Note close relationship of megakaryocytes to reticulin
fibers. (Gordon-Sweets', ×530.)

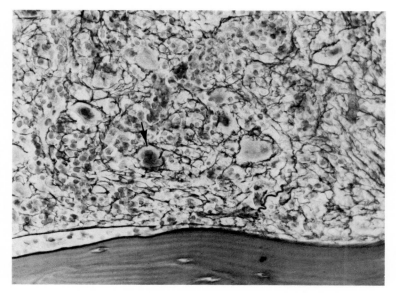

Figure 4-17
Agnogenic myeloid metaplasia. Note reticulin myelofibrosis (see p. 153) and
increased number of megakaryocytes. The megakaryocytes are surrounded by
reticulin fibers (*arrow*). (Gordon-Sweets', ×160.)

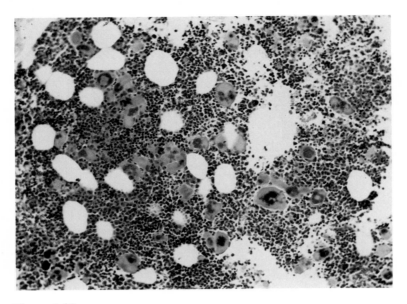

Figure 4-18
Essential thrombocythemia. Increased megakaryocytes with preservation of fat cells. (H&E, ×114.)

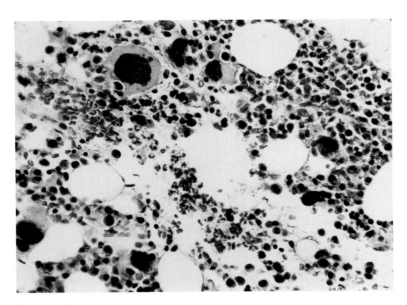

Figure 4-19
Megakaryocytic myelosis. Note cytologically atypical megakaryocytes. (H&E, ×308.)

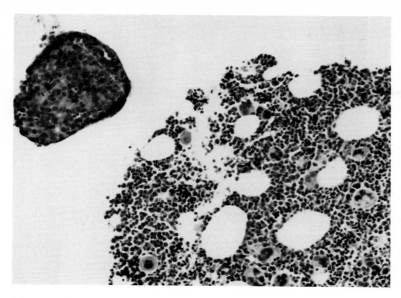

Figure 4-20
Increased megakaryocytes in metastatic carcinoma (*left upper corner*). (H&E, ×132.)

fying thrombocytic and megakaryocytic myelosis." Occasionally, mega-karyocytic hyperplasia is observed in association with metastatic carcinoma (Fig. 4-20).

References

1. Crosby, W. H.   Wet purpura, dry purpura. *J.A.M.A.* 232:744, 1975.
2. Di Guglielmo, G.   L'erythromégakaryocytémie aiguë. *Sang* 27:671, 1956.
3. Franzen, S., Strenger, G., and Zajicek, J.   Microplanimetric studies on megakaryocytes in chronic granulocytic leukemia and polycythemia vera. *Acta Haematol.* 26:182, 1961.
4. Guichard, A., Fayelle, J., Alex, R., and Revol, J.   Myélose aleucémique décalcifiante à plaquettes et à mégacaryocytes: La leucémie à plaquettes. *Sang* 27:337, 1956.
5. Lagerlof, B.   Cytophotometric study of megakaryocyte ploidy in polycythemia vera and chronic granulocytic leukemia. *Acta Cytol.* 16:240, 1972.
6. McDonald, J. B., and Hamrick, J. G.   Acute megakaryocytic leukemia. *Arch. Intern. Med.* 81:73, 1948.
7. Rappaport, H.   Tumors of the Hematopoietic System. In *Atlas of Tumor Pathology*. Washington, D.C.: Armed Forces Institute of Pathology, 1966. Sect. III, Fasc. 8, p. 295.

5 The Red Cell Series

Normoblastic Maturation

The maturation of the red cell series may be normoblastic or megaloblastic. Normoblastic maturation, which is the normal maturation, is easily recognized in hematoxylin and eosin-stained sections of aspirated bone marrow particles. The normoblasts are arranged in groups and exhibit perfectly round, homogeneous, darkly basophilic nuclei (Fig. 5-1). The nuclei are relatively pyknotic, and little nuclear detail can be made out. The size of the nuclei and their degree of pyknosis depend on the maturity of the normoblast—the more mature the cell, the smaller and more pyknotic is the nucleus. Often the normoblastic nuclei are completely surrounded by a halo apparently caused by an artifactual retraction of the cytoplasm (Fig. 5-2). The cytoplasm of the mature normoblasts is difficult to see in histologic sections. The hematoxylin and eosin stain allows recognition of mature (orthochromatic) normoblasts, but it is not a good stain for basophilic normoblasts. It is much easier to recognize the latter with the Giemsa stain, which brings out the basophilia of the cytoplasm. Pronormoblasts (rubriblasts, proerythroblasts, erythroblasts) are recognized by their larger nuclei, which are perfectly round, contain prominent nucleoli, and are surrounded by a dark blue rim of cytoplasm made prominent by the Giemsa stain. They are distinguished from basophilic normoblasts by their larger nuclei and the presence of nucleoli. Pronormoblasts are distinguished from other blasts by the company they keep—that is, by their association with more mature nucleated red blood cells—and by the more intense basophilia of their cytoplasm.

Beginners in the study of histologic sections of bone marrow may find it difficult to distinguish between normoblasts and lymphocytes. Lymphocytes occur in the marrow in nodules that are much more discrete than normoblastic groups and that are easily recognized under low magnification (see Chap. 9). Furthermore, the lymphocytic nuclei are not as perfectly round as those of normoblasts, and they show more variability in size and shape. More intranuclear detail is seen in lymphocytic than in normoblastic nuclei. In addition, the perinuclear halo of normoblasts is helpful in distinguishing them from lymphocytes (see Fig. 5-2).

Numerical Considerations

In anemias the number of nucleated red cells in the bone marrow may be increased or decreased. Though considerable numerical data are available on differential counts of bone marrow smears, very little work has been done on quantitating nucleated red cells in histologic sections.

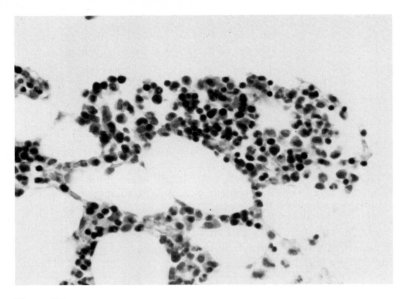

Figure 5-1
Appearance of normoblasts in sections. Note almost perfectly round, pyknotic nuclei. (H&E, ×416.)

No data are available as to how many nucleated red blood cells are present in the normoblastic nests in normal marrows. Extreme degrees of erythroblastic (normoblastic or erythroid) hyperplasia or hypoplasia can be easily recognized. Minor deviations are more difficult to appreciate. Perhaps the best way for the morphologic quantitative evaluation of erythropoiesis is to estimate the relative numbers of nucleated red blood cells and granulocytes. Normally, as in smears, there are considerably more granulocytes than nucleated red blood cells. However, the ratio of granulocytes to nucleated red blood cells is not as high in histologic sections prepared by our technic as in smears, because of the loss of some granulocytes in the filtering process when the bone marrow particles are concentrated. Thus the normal ratio of granulocytes to nucleated red cells in histologic sections is from 2:1 to 3:1. A decrease in this ratio may mean that there is erythroblastic hyperplasia or granulocytic hypoplasia and thus an absolute or a relative erythroblastic hyperplasia. To decide whether absolute or relative hyperplasia is present, the above ratio has to be evaluated in conjunction with the general cellularity of the marrow.

Erythroblastic hyperplasia (erythroid hyperplasia) may be normoblastic or megaloblastic in maturation. It can be seen with many different hematologic conditions (see following list).

Erythroblastic Hyperplasia (*normoblastic or megaloblastic*)

Iron deficiency anemia
Hemolytic anemias
Refractory anemias with hypercellular marrows
Megaloblastic anemias
Polycythemia vera
Hypoxia
Erythroblastic hyperplasia with refractory anemia caused by giant lymph
    node hyperplasia [6, 7]
Erythrocytosis associated with neoplasms or renal disease
Dyserythropoiesis
    Erythroleukemia
    Erythremic myelosis
    Congenital dyserythropoietic anemias

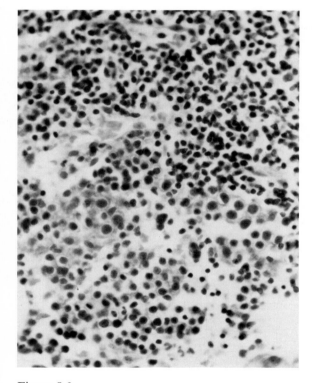

Figure 5-2
Sheet of macronormoblasts below lymphoid nodule. Note perfectly round
nuclei and perinuclear halo of nucleated red blood cells (*lower half of photo-
graph*). The nucleated red cells are somewhat larger than normal (see Fig.
5-1). (H&E, ×416.)

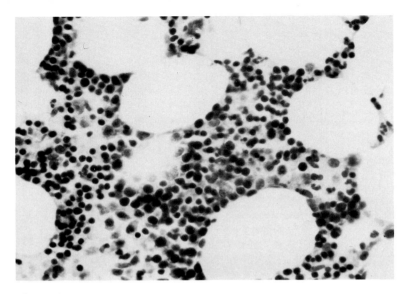

Figure 5-3
Moderately severe erythroblastic hyperplasia. Note predominance of nucleated red blood cells and good preservation of fat cells. (H&E, ×416.)

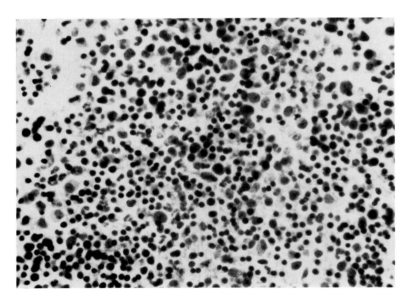

Figure 5-4
Very severe erythroblastic hyperplasia in a patient with thalassemia. Note hypercellularity of marrow with disappearance of fat cells. (H&E, ×438.)

The degree of erythroblastic hyperplasia seems to depend on the severity of the anemia and on the ability of the marrow to respond to erythropoietin. Erythroblastic hyperplasia may be associated with effective or ineffective erythropoiesis. In ineffective erythropoiesis, relatively few red cells reach the peripheral blood even though there is considerable erythroblastic hyperplasia.

Erythroblastic hyperplasia is more marked in hemolytic anemias than in iron deficiency anemia. With marked erythroblastic hyperplasia, the red cell series exhibits a shift to the left with the appearance of an increased number of pronormoblasts. Megaloblastoid features may appear, perhaps because of a relative folic acid deficiency caused by the intense proliferation of red blood cell precursors. Examples of erythroblastic hyperplasia are shown in Figures 5-3 and 5-4. In Figure 5-4 the erythroblastic hyperplasia is so severe that it has replaced the normal fat cells of the marrow.

Erythroblastic hypoplasia is seen in conjunction with general marrow hypoplasia involving also the granulocytic and megakaryocytic series. It may also occur in a "pure" form in which the hypoplasia is limited to the red cell series. The term *aplastic anemia* is often applied to patients with refractory anemia and pancytopenia, regardless of whether the marrow is actually hypocellular or hypercellular. Conditions that may cause erythroblastic hypoplasia are cited in the following list.

Erythroblastic Hypoplasia
(May be "pure," i.e., limited to red cell series, or part of general marrow hypoplasia)

Congenital hypoplastic anemia
    Fanconi's anemia (familial constitutional panmyelocytopathy) [4]
    Familial hypoplastic anemia of Estren and Dameshek [3]
Idiopathic aplastic anemia
Chemicals and drugs
Radiation
"Pure" erythroblastic hypoplasia (pure red cell aplasia)
    Congenital: Diamond-Blackfan type [1]
    Related to thymoma (spindle cell type)
    Idiopathic
    Aplastic crises in hemolytic anemias
    Drugs
Paroxysmal nocturnal hemoglobinuria
Preleukemia
Viral infections and tuberculosis

Megaloblastic Maturation

The term *megaloblast* does not refer to one specific type of red cell. It denotes any maturation stage of a megaloblastic red cell series. Thus there is a promegaloblast, a basophilic megaloblast, a polychromato-philic megaloblast, an orthochromatic megaloblast, and an adult mega-locyte or macrocyte. The term *megaloblastic maturation* is not limited to the red cell series. It is also applied to granulocytic and megakaryocytic maturation.

Megaloblastic maturation is more difficult to recognize in histologic sections than in bone marrow smears. The marrow is usually markedly hypercellular and diffusely infiltrated with cells which at first glance resemble histiocytes or reticulum cells (Fig. 5-5). More detailed obser-vation, however, reveals that the nuclei are perfectly round, remarkably uniform, and centrally located in the cytoplasm. If one then looks for fully hemoglobinized nucleated red blood cells, they are much larger than those seen in normoblastic maturation. Also, contrary to normo-blastic maturation, the orthochromatic cytoplasm of megaloblasts is easily recognized, even with medium power magnification (Figs. 5-5 to 5-7). In Giemsa-stained sections the more immature megaloblasts are distinguished from reticulum cells or macrophages by their dark blue rim of cytoplasm (Fig. 5-8). The immature megaloblasts have to be identified as erythroid cells in order to avoid an erroneous diagnosis of an acute blastic leukemia.

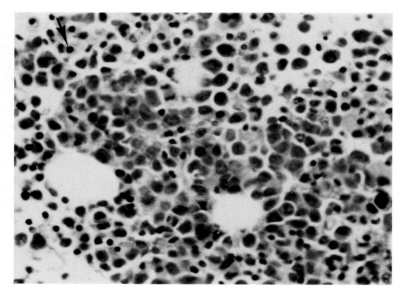

Figure 5-5
Megaloblastic erythropoiesis. Note larger size, prominent nucleoli, and rela-tive pallor of nuclei when compared to normoblastic erythropoiesis. Note orthochromatic megaloblasts with slightly eccentric, pyknotic nucleus and relatively abundant cytoplasm (*arrow*). (H&E, ×416.)

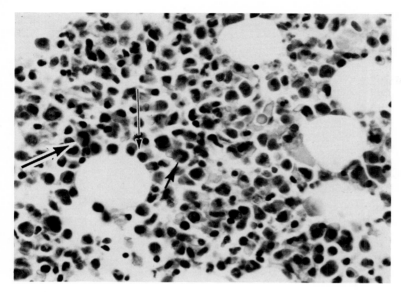

Figure 5-6
Megaloblastic erythropoiesis. Note abundant cytoplasm in late (orthochromatic) megaloblast (*thin black-and-white arrow*). In late normoblasts the cytoplasm is difficult to see in formalin-fixed, Paraplast-embedded sections. Also note giant band (*black arrow*) and giant metamyelocyte (*broad black-and-white arrow*). (H&E, ×416.)

Megaloblastic maturation affects all the red cell precursors but is easiest to recognize in the megaloblastic polychromatophilic and orthochromatic nucleated red blood cells (Fig. 5-7). Confirmatory evidence of a megaloblastic maturation can also be obtained from a search for giant metamyelocytes and hypersegmented polymorphonuclear leukocytes and megakaryocytes (Fig. 5-6).

Megaloblastic or normoblastic maturation is not an all-or-none phenomenon, and intermediate stages of red cell maturation can be seen. These are referred to as *megaloblastoid* or *macronormoblastic maturation* (see Fig. 5-2). The nucleated red cells in this type of maturation are intermediate in size and nuclear features between the characteristic normoblastic and megaloblastic appearances. Macronormoblastic or megaloblastoid features may be focal in distribution—that is, they may present in one bone marrow particle and not in others—or they may be seen in only some red cell clumps. This intermediate type of maturation may be seen in folic acid deficiency, liver disease, and hemolytic and sideroblastic anemias.

Causes of megaloblastic maturation are summarized in the following list.

Pernicious anemia
Congenital intrinsic factor deficiency
Congenital vitamin B_{12} malabsorption
Dietary deficiency of vitamin B_{12} (strict vegetarians)
Nutritional folate deficiency
Gastrectomy
Gut resection and malabsorption
Abnormal intestinal bacterial flora (blind loop, diverticula, fistulae, strictures)
Fish tapeworm
Megaloblastic anemia of pregnancy
Drugs (anticonvulsants, folate antagonists)
Megaloblastosis secondary to blood disorders (hemolytic anemias, sideroblastic anemias, leukemias)
Miscellaneous (orotic acid aciduria, hemochromatosis)

It has to be emphasized that a diagnosis of pernicious anemia cannot be made with certainty from the bone marrow alone. Only a diagnosis of megaloblastic maturation can be made, and other studies are necessary to establish the cause of the megaloblastosis. Pernicious anemia can be suspected on morphologic grounds alone when the marrow is markedly

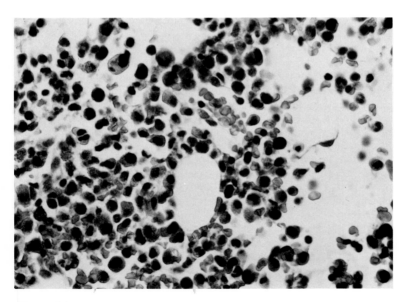

Figure 5-7
Megaloblastic erythropoiesis. Note numerous late megaloblasts with pyknotic, large nuclei and relatively abundant cytoplasm. (H&E, ×416.)

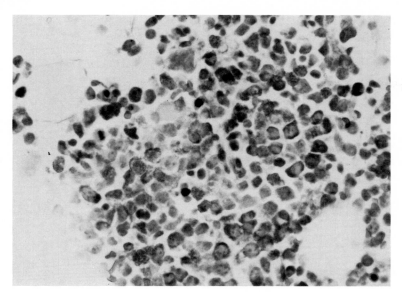

Figure 5-8
Megaloblastic erythropoiesis. Note predominance of basophilic megaloblasts with dark blue rims of cytoplasm and large nuclei with prominent nucleoli. This picture can be confused with an acute blastic leukemia unless the erythroid nature of the blasts is recognized. (Giemsa, ×453.)

hypercellular and shows full-blown megaloblastic features in all three cell series.

Dyserythropoiesis

Dyserythropoiesis refers to varying degrees of cellular atypism in the nucleated red blood cells. It generally is associated with erythroblastic hyperplasia and with at least some megaloblastoid features (Fig. 5-9). The red cells are enlarged and show large, hyperchromatic, bizarre nuclei. Binucleated or multinucleated red blood cells may be present. Conditions associated with dyserythropoiesis are tabulated in the list on page 50.

Neoplastic-appearing erythroblasts, both normoblastic and megaloblastoid, may appear in sheets replacing fat cells. If this marked proliferation of atypical erythroblasts is associated with a proliferation of myeloblasts, one is justified in diagnosing erythroleukemia (see Fig. 5-9). As the disease progresses the marrow takes on the appearance of an acute blastic leukemia.

Occasionally, a definite increase in myeloblasts is difficult to demonstrate and the bone marrow is profusely crowded with markedly atypical nucleated red bood cells in the presence of normally maturing granulo-

Congenital dyserythropoietic anemias [5]
  Type I—autosomal recessive
  (megaloblastoid red cells with internuclear chromatin bridges)
  Type II—autosomal recessive [2]
  (HEMPAS—*H*ereditary *E*rythroblastic *M*ultinuclearity with *P*ositive *A*cid *S*erum test. Also Gaucher-like cells and agglutination by anti-i serum)
  Type III—autosomal dominant
  (enlarged multinucleated erythroblasts)
Erythroleukemia and erythremic myelosis
Some refractory anemias
Preleukemic state
Pernicious anemia

cytes (Fig. 5-10). This appearance of the bone marrow is associated with a marked increase in atypical nucleated red blood cells in the peripheral blood. The term *erythremic myelosis* has been applied to this invariably fatal disease. An acute and a chronic form have been recog-

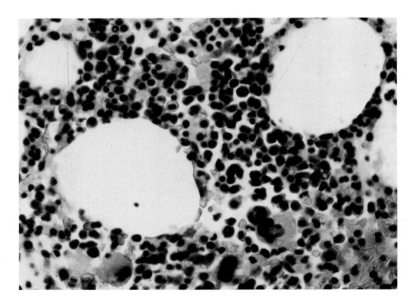

Figure 5-9
Dyserythropoiesis in erythroleukemia. Erythroblastic hyperplasia, variability in nuclear size and shape of red blood cells, and relatively abundant cytoplasm of orthochromatic red blood cells reflecting their megaloblastoid maturation. Note absence of mature granulocytes. (H&E, ×451.)

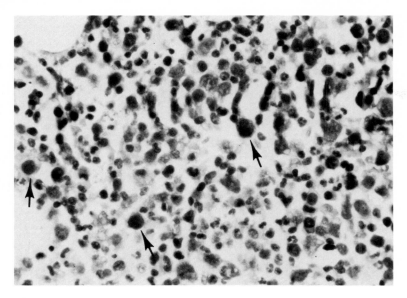

Figure 5-10
Erythremic myelosis. Markedly atypical, large, nucleated red blood cells (*arrows*) with normal maturation of granulocytes. (H&E, ×416.)

nized. The acute form is characterized by a more rapid course, by more immature erythroblasts in the peripheral blood, and by greater atypism of the erythroblasts in the bone marrow.

A number of diseases have to be considered in the differential diagnosis of a bone marrow exhibiting a markedly atypical erythroblastic hyperplasia. In pernicious anemia there may be marked atypism of the nucleated red cells, and it is occasionally difficult to distinguish it from erythremic myelosis. The nucleated red blood cells in erythremic myelosis may contain glycogen, which can be demonstrated with the PAS stain. Because glycogen is water soluble and formalin is an aqueous fixative, it is easier to demonstrate the glycogen in smears fixed in absolute alcohol. When there is the slightest doubt whether a patient has pernicious anemia or an erythremic myelosis, it is best to submit the patient to a trial of vitamin B_{12} and folic acid therapy before a definitive diagnosis is made. Other laboratory tests such as vitamin B_{12} levels and the Schilling test are also useful.

The congenital dyserythropoietic anemias show marked erythroblastic hyperplasia with atypism and can be mistaken for erythremic myelosis (see list). In type I there are rather characteristic internuclear chromatin bridges in the abnormal erythroblasts. Patients with type II dyserythropoietic anemia may exhibit Gaucher-like cells in their marrow (see Chap. 10).

Some of the refractory anemias with hypercellular marrow may also mimic erythremic myelosis. The demonstration of numerous ringed sideroblasts and the absence of PAS-positive material in the erythroblasts may help in the differential diagnosis (see Plate IB). Refractory anemias may also exhibit a marked increase in megakaryocytes and mast cells. Sideroblastic anemias are discussed in more detail in Chapter 6.

References

1. Diamond, L. K., and Blackfan, K. D. Hypoplastic anemia. *Am. J. Dis. Child.* 56:464, 1938.
2. Enquist, R. W., Gockerman, J. P., Jenis, E. H., Warkel, R. L., and Dillon, D. E. Type II congenital dyserythropoietic anemia. *Ann. Intern. Med.* 77:371, 1972.
3. Estren, S., and Dameshek, W. Familial hypoplastic anemia of childhood: Report of eight cases in two families with beneficial effect of splenectomy in one case. *Am. J. Dis. Child.* 73:671, 1947.
4. Fanconi, G. Familial constitutional panmyelocytopathy, Fanconi's anemia. *Semin. Hematol.* 4:233, 1967.
5. Heimpel, H., and Wendt, E. Congenital dyserythropoietic anemia with karyorrhexis and multinuclearity of erythroblasts. *Helv. Med. Acta* 34:103, 1968.
6. Keller, H. R., Hochholzer, L., and Castleman, B. Hyaline-vascular and plasma cell types of giant lymph node hyperplasia of the mediastinum and other locations. *Cancer* 29:670, 1972.
7. Lee, S. L., Rosner, F., Rivero, I., Feldman, F., and Hurwitz, A. Refractory anemia with abnormal metabolism: Its remission after resection of hyperplastic mediastinal lymph nodes. *N. Engl. J. Med.* 272:761, 1965.

6 Bone Marrow Hemosiderin

Terminology and Technics

The total-body elemental iron content of a normal adult is 3 to 5 gm. About 25 percent of the iron is in storage almost equally divided between ferritin and hemosiderin. It is estimated that one-third of the storage iron is found in the bone marrow [10]. Ferritin is composed of a protein, apoferritin, in which are held ferric hydroxide micelles. Ferritin, which is very finely dispersed within the cytoplasm, is not visible with the light microscope. It is water soluble and is removed to some extent by aqueous fixatives such as formalin.

Hemosiderin seems to be formed gradually as the ferritin molecules age and aggregate into yellow to brown granules visible with the light microscope. The apoferritin molecules are partially denatured with a resulting increase in iron content of hemosiderin as compared to ferritin.

Bone marrow hemosiderin content (iron stores) is evaluated on the basis of a histochemical reaction between the ferric iron of hemosiderin and an acid solution of potassium ferrocyanide. This results in the formation of ferri-ferrocyanide, $Fe_4[Fe(CN)_6]_3$, also known as Prussian blue (see Appendix, 2). Only the ferric iron of hemosiderin participates in this reaction, so that hemosiderin granules appear as dark blue, intracellular granules of varying sizes. The ferric iron of the ferritin does not participate in the Prussian blue reaction. This is not due to the solubility of ferritin in aqueous fixatives, because fixation in absolute alcohol does not bring out the ferritin either. Fixation in 10% neutral buffered formalin actually gives the best Prussian blue reaction [7]. Perhaps ferritin does not react with potassium ferrocyanide because it is too finely dispersed in the cytoplasm. It is possible, however, that the fine diffuse staining occasionally seen in histiocytes and attributed by Lillie to protosiderin [7] is actually due to ferritin or a transition substance between ferritin and hemosiderin. It has been shown that the diffuse bluish hue of Gaucher's cells stained by the Prussian blue procedure is due to an increased amount of finely dispersed ferritin [8].

The evaluation of iron stores in unstained smears is not reliable, because hemosiderin cannot be unequivocally distinguished from other brown pigments such as melanin, malarial pigment, or ceroid.

When the histologist describes "iron stores" he means hemosiderin content, and it would be more appropriate to speak of hemosiderin granules rather than of iron stores. It should also be remembered that bone marrow hemosiderin does not necessarily reflect hemosiderin deposits in other organs. Thus in paroxysmal nocturnal hemoglobinuria the bone marrow hemosiderin content may be depleted in the presence of renal hemosiderosis. Similarly, in idiopathic pulmonary siderosis the lungs are filled with hemosiderin, whereas the hemosiderin content of the bone marrow may be depleted. Serum ferritin levels seem to correlate well with bone marrow hemosiderin [2].

Section versus Smear

The Prussian blue reaction can be applied to histologic sections as well as to smears of bone marrow. Both sections and smears yield reliable results, though discrepancies between the two are occasionally noted. Adequate smears for evaluation of hemosiderin content have to be relatively thick and must contain crushed particles, for the latter contain the histiocytes with the hemosiderin granules. Sections are much thinner and permit the intracellular location of the hemosiderin granules to be ascertained. Prussian blue preparations, whether sections or smears, often contain extracellular blue precipitates that represent artifacts and should not be misread as hemosiderin, which can be recognized with certainty only when it is intracellular. Artifacts are easier to recognize in sections than in smears.

Discrepancies between sections and smears in the evaluation of hemosiderin content have been reported in 16 percent of cases [9]. Lundin et al. [9] have pointed out that the absence of hemosiderin must be evaluated in relation to the quantity of marrow examined and that this evaluation can be performed with more confidence when sections are used.

Morphology

Hemosiderin granules appear in the bone marrow in reticulum cells, macrophages, endothelial cells, and red cells. In reticulum cells they appear as granules of varying size, which may form clumps (Plate IA, B). The hemosiderin granules usually fill the reticulum cell completely and outline the elongated, somewhat stellate shape of the cytoplasm. Hemosiderin granules can be easily recognized in hematoxylin and eosin-stained sections as yellow to brown granules, which become refractile when the iris diaphragm is narrowed or the condenser lowered. This observation of hemosiderin in hematoxylin and eosin-stained sections serves as a partial control for the Prussian blue reaction. However, as with every special stain, a positive control slide should be stained. It has been said that in hemochromatosis the hemosiderin granules have a finely particulate appearance which contrasts with the hemosiderin clumps seen in transfusion hemosiderosis [3].

Patients who have received iron-dextran injections, or who have increased hemosiderin content from excessive ingestion of iron salts, also exhibit finely particulate "hemosiderin" granules [3]. Because these granules are not derived from red blood cells, *siderin* granules is a more accurate term. The "amorphous" hemosiderin deposits described by Wallerstein and Pollycove [14] as characteristics of patients with aplastic anemia may represent confluent hemosiderin granules. A more likely explanation is that these "amorphous" deposits which stain the cytoplasm diffusely, and which are paler than the granular hemosiderin, are related to what Lillie [7] has called protosiderin, probably a transition stage between ferritin and hemosiderin. Occasionally, hemosiderin granules are found in endothelial cells (Plate IA). There is no direct relationship between the hemosiderin content of reticulum cells and histologically observable erythrophagocytosis.

Hemosiderin granules are also present in nucleated and mature red cells. They are much smaller than the granules in reticulum cells. Nucleated red cells containing hemosiderin are called *sideroblasts*. *Siderocytes* are anuclear red cells with tiny hemosiderin granules. Normal sideroblasts and siderocytes are easier to see in smears than in sections. Ringed sideroblasts are characteristic of sideroblastic anemias. Their hemosiderin granules are considerably larger than in normal sideroblasts and form a perinuclear ring. They are easily seen in both smears and sections (Plate IB).

Quantitative Considerations

Hemosiderin may be distributed fairly uniformly in different bone marrow particles, or it may show a spotty distribution with no hemosiderin in some particles and varying amounts in others. This irregular distribution has to be kept in mind, and the diagnosis of depleted hemosiderin content on the basis of an examination of a single bone marrow particle is not appropriate.

No exact quantitative data are available as to what, histochemically, constitutes a normal amount of bone marrow hemosiderin. Absence or a marked decrease of hemosiderin granules, as well as a marked increase, are easily recognized. The precise limits between normal and a slight decrease or increase of hemosiderin are ill defined. For this reason the terms suggested for the description of bone marrow hemosiderin are (1) absent or markedly decreased; (2) present; or (3) increased. Little additional information seems to be gained by quantitating the hemosiderin from 0 to 4+ or 6+ by different criteria, usually relying on how many oil-immersion fields contain hemosiderin granules [3].

In our experience the counting of sideroblasts is of little practical value. In general, when the marrow contains very little or no hemosiderin, sideroblasts are decreased or absent. After an acute hemorrhage, there may be no sideroblasts in the marrow in the presence of normal hemosiderin content [3]. On the other hand, during the treatment of iron deficiency anemia, the sideroblast count of the marrow may become normal whereas the hemosiderin content of the marrow is still depleted [4]. The sideroblast count does not appear to show any consistent increase with iron excess [1].

Decreased or Depleted Bone Marrow Hemosiderin

The conditions giving rise to decreased or depleted hemosiderin content follow.

Physiologic state (e.g.: newborn)
Some asymptomatic, nonanemic patients
Iron deficiency anemia
Paroxysmal nocturnal hemoglobinuria
Idiopathic pulmonary hemosiderosis
Intravascular hemolysis with hemosiderinuria
    Anemia associated with prosthetic heart valves
Congenital hypotransferrinemia or atransferrinemia
Congenital iron deficiency anemia with hyperferremia [12]
Some megaloblastic anemias (dimorphic anemia)
Some cases of anemia with giant lymph node hyperplasia [6]

Iron deficiency anemia is usually hypochromic and microcytic. Early in the development of the anemia it may be normochromic and normocytic.

In exceptional cases a hypochromic, microcytic anemia caused by iron deficiency may be observed in the presence of bone marrow hemosiderin or "siderin." This occurs after recent administration of iron-dextran, saccharated iron oxide, or even blood transfusions. Parenterally administered iron appears not to be as readily available for erythropoiesis as normally occurring hemosiderin [3].

Hypochromic, microcytic anemia may also be seen in association with normal or increased bone marrow hemosiderin, seen in the thalassemias, pyridoxine responsive anemia, hereditary sideroblastic anemia, lead poisoning, and other anemias in which iron cannot be properly utilized, such as the anemia of chronic infection.

Increased Bone Marrow Hemosiderin

As a rule the hemosiderin content is increased in all anemias other than those appearing in the preceding list. The iron not utilized for the red cell pool is shifted to the stores. In intravascular hemolytic processes there is hemosiderinuria and depletion of iron stores. In extravascular hemolysis or ineffective erythropoiesis (intramedullary hemolysis) there is an increase in hemosiderin content.

Hemosiderin content is increased in patients with hemochromatosis and hemosiderosis (see list on p. 57).

Idiopathic or primary hemochromatosis is a disease of debated etiology and pathogenesis characterized by an excessive accumulation of hemosiderin and other pigments, accompanied by cirrhosis of the liver and often fibrosis of the pancreas. The hemosiderin content of the bone marrow is markedly and diffusely increased. Fibrosis of the marrow is not generally seen. The hemosiderin is said to be distributed in relatively fine particles [1].

Secondary hemochromatosis occurs in patients with long-standing hemolytic anemia with erythroblastic hyperplasia of the bone marrow.

Anemias other than those listed previously
Sideroblastic anemias (see following list)
Erythremic myelosis
Idiopathic or primary hemochromatosis
Secondary hemochromatosis
Hemosiderosis
Some cases of portacaval shunt siderosis [13]
Bantu siderosis (?)
Porphyria cutanea tarda (?)

Often there is a history of numerous transfusions and/or prolonged administration of iron salts. The bone marrow hemosiderin is similar to that in primary hemochromatosis.

Siderosis and even a hemochromatosis-like picture have been described in patients following portacaval end-to-side anastomosis for bleeding varices in cirrhosis of the liver [13]. Though the liver contains an increased amount of hemosiderin in this condition, the bone marrow usually has normal or even depleted hemosiderin content. Some patients, however, have increased bone marrow hemosiderin.

Sideroblastic Anemias

The sideroblastic anemias (see following list) include a group of disorders characterized by a chronic anemia associated with bone marrow findings, including (1) hypercellular marrow with erythroblastic hyperplasia, (2) increased marrow hemosiderin, and (3) the presence of numerous ringed sideroblasts.

Sideroblastic Anemias

Primary
    Acquired
    Hereditary, sex-linked
Pyridoxine-responsive
Secondary
    Sideroblastic anemia associated with a variety of hematologic, neoplastic, and collagen vascular diseases
    Drug-induced
    Lead poisoning

The etiology and pathogenesis of these anemias is not well understood, but there is evidence that at least in some of them there is a disturbance in heme synthesis. This is certainly not true for thalassemia, in which there is a disturbance in globin synthesis, though on the basis of the above criteria thalassemia can be placed in the group of sideroblastic anemias. In the sideroblastic anemias, ringed sideroblasts are abundant (Plate IB). Rare ringed sideroblasts can occasionally be found in the marrow of patients with other conditions. The significance of this finding is unknown. The cases of erythroleukemia associated with ringed sideroblasts may well have evolved from primary acquired sideroblastic anemias. The positive PAS staining of the normoblastic cytoplasm in erythroleukemia is helpful in confirming the diagnosis. However, a PAS-positive reaction of normoblasts has been reported in thalassemia [11] and in chronic renal disease [5].

Some patients with primary acquired sideroblastic anemia exhibit megaloblastoid erythropoiesis. In addition the nucleated red cells may exhibit considerable atypism, and megakaryocytes and mast cells may be increased.

References

1. Beutler, E.   Clinical evaluation of iron stores. *N. Engl. J. Med.* 256:692, 1957.
2. Editorial.   Serum-ferritin. *Lancet* 1:1263, 1974.
3. Fairbanks, V. F., Fahey, J. L., and Beutler, E.   *Clinical Disorders of Iron Metabolism* (2nd ed.). New York: Grune & Stratton, 1971. Pp. 196, 421.
4. Hansen, H. A., and Weinfeld, A.   Hemosiderin estimations and sideroblast counts in the differential diagnosis of iron deficiency and other anemias. *Acta Med. Scand.* 165:333, 1959.
5. Klein, H. O., and Heller, A.   PAS-positive erythroblasts in kidney diseases. *Acta Haematol.* 37:225, 1967.
6. Lee, S. L., Rosner, F., Rivero, I., Feldman, F., and Hurwitz, A.   Refractory anemia with abnormal iron metabolism: Its remission after resection of hyperplastic mediastinal lymph nodes. *N. Engl. J. Med.* 272:761, 1965.
7. Lillie, R. D.   *Histopathologic Technic and Practical Histochemistry* (3rd ed.). New York: Blakiston Div., McGraw-Hill, 1965. Pp. 401, 403.
8. Lorber, M.   Adult-type Gaucher's disease: A secondary disorder of iron metabolism. *J. Mt. Sinai Hosp.* 37:404, 1970.
9. Lundin, P., Persson, E., and Weinfeld, A.   Comparison of hemosiderin estimation in bone marrow sections and bone marrow smears. *Acta Med. Scand.* 175:383, 1964.
10. Pollycove, M.   Iron metabolism and kinetics. *Semin. Hematol.* 3:235, 1966.
11. Quaglino, D., and Hayhoe, F. G.   Periodic-acid-Schiff positivity in erythroblasts with special reference to di Guglielmo's disease. *Br. J. Haematol.* 6:26, 1960.
12. Shahidi, N. T., Nathan, D. G., and Diamond, L. K.   Iron deficiency anemia associated with an error of iron metabolism in two siblings. *J. Clin. Invest.* 43:510, 1964.
13. Tisdale, W. A.   Parenchymal siderosis in patients with cirrhosis after portasystemic shunt surgery. *N. Engl. J. Med.* 265:928, 1961.
14. Wallerstein, R. O., and Pollycove, M.   Bone marrow hemosiderin and ferrokinetics patterns in anemia. *Arch. Intern. Med.* 101:418, 1958.

7 Granulocytes

Six maturation stages are recognized in granulopoiesis as observed in Romanovsky-stained bone marrow smears: myeloblast, promyelocyte, myelocyte, metamyelocyte, band granulocyte, and mature polymorphonuclear leukocyte. Mature granulocytes are easily recognized in histologic sections of aspirated bone marrow particles. The linear nuclear bridges linking the lobes of a fully segmented granulocyte are not seen in histologic sections. The nucleus of the mature granulocyte looks as if it were composed of small nuclear lobes touching each other (Fig. 7-1). Band granulocytes can be recognized even under relatively low magnification because of their characteristically horseshoe-shaped nucleus (Fig. 7-1). Frequently histologic sections of bone marrows rich in granulocytes contain small collections of granular hematoxylinophilic debris derived from granulocytic nuclei (Fig. 7-2). This debris should not be mistaken for bacteria or parasites. Myelocytes, promyelocytes, and myeloblasts are difficult to identify with certainty in hematoxylin and eosin-stained sections of formalin-fixed bone marrow. In bone marrow particles fixed in Zenker's solution more nuclear detail is seen, so that myelocytes can be distinguished from promyelocytes and myeloblasts by their heavier nuclear chromatin. In formalin-fixed, hematoxylin and eosin-stained sections the specific granules of neutrophilic granulocytes can be perceived when the iris diaphragm is narrowed. Myelocytes can be identified with ease in Paraplast-embedded sections of formalin-fixed tissue by means of the Leder stain (see Appendix, 5) [2]. In the Leder reaction neutrophilic and mast cell granules are stained selectively red (Plate IC, D). The stain is based on the presence in the granules of an esterase that reacts with a substrate consisting of a substituted naphthol acetate (naphthol ASD). The Leder reaction does not stain eosinophilic granules. Myeloblasts can be recognized with the Giemsa stain, which gives good results with formalin-fixed embedded tissues. Like all blasts the myeloblasts exhibit a rim of blue cytoplasm, but less intense than that of proerythroblasts. The nucleus has distinct nucleoli. Promyelocytes cannot be recognized accurately, because azurophilic granules are not demonstrated in tissue sections. Neutrophilic granules can also be stained in embedded tissue sections with the PAS reaction (see Appendix, 7), with Sudan black, and with Goodpasture's peroxidase stain. In practice, special stains other than the Leder and Giemsa stains are rarely necessary.

Polymorphonuclear leukocytes have a peculiar attraction for megakaryocytes and for platelets. Often polymorphonuclear leukocytes surround a megakaryocyte or a fragment of megakaryocytic cytoplasm (Fig. 7-3). When there is increased platelet production, peculiar ring-shaped or serpentine platelet aggregates are formed which are sur-

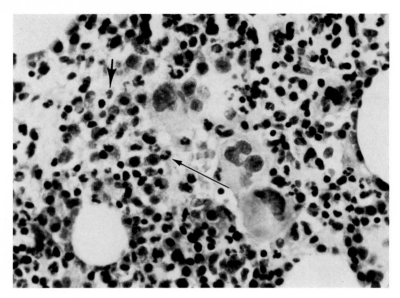

Figure 7-1
Appearance of mature, fully segmented granulocytes (*long arrow*). They are recognized by their nuclei, which appear to be made up of small nuclear lobes touching each other. Band granulocytes have a horseshoe-shaped nucleus (*short arrow*). Also note megakaryocytes and nucleated red cells (H&E, ×416.)

rounded by a layer of polymorphonuclear leukocytes (Fig. 7-4; see Fig. 4-5).

Giant metamyelocytes and hypersegmented polymorphonuclear leukocytes are easily seen in histologic sections. Giant metamyelocytes can be spotted under relatively low magnification (Fig. 7-5). Romanovsky-stained smears are necessary for the identification of toxic granulations, Döhle's inclusion bodies, and the May-Hegglin and Alder anomalies. Pelger-Huët cells and the Chédiak-Higashi anomaly are easier to recognize in smears than in sections.

Granulocytic Hyperplasia and Leukemoid Reactions

The normal marrow contains more granulocytes than nucleated red blood cells. In histologic sections the granulocyte (myeloid) to nucleated red blood cell (erythroid) ratio (M:E ratio) varies from 2:1 to 3:1. Granulocytic hyperplasia is present when this ratio is exceeded in a hypercellular marrow. The M:E ratio alone cannot define granulocytic hyperplasia because it can be increased in erythroid hypoplasia. By convention, granulocytic hyperplasia and hypoplasia refer to neutrophils and their precursors (promyelocytes and myeloblasts) which do not contain

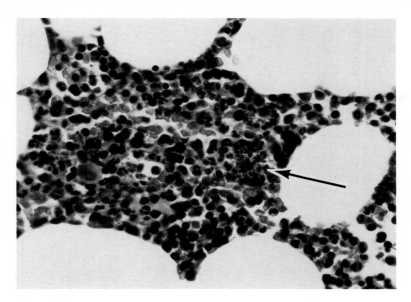

Figure 7-2
Granulocytic debris (*arrow*). This appears to be an artifact resulting from granulocytic fragmentation and aggregation. (H&E, ×466).

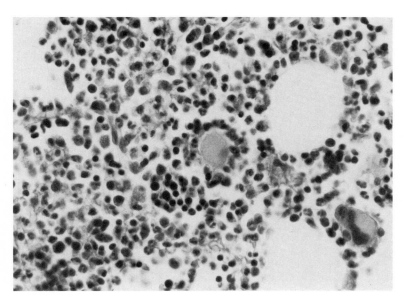

Figure 7-3
Megakaryocyte surrounded by polymorphonuclear leukocytes. (H&E, ×416.)

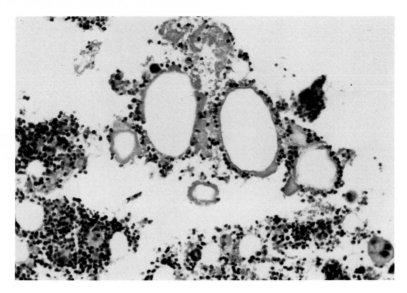

Figure 7-4
Ring-shaped structures composed of platelets and adherent polymorphonuclear leukocytes (see also Fig. 4-5). (H&E, ×162.)

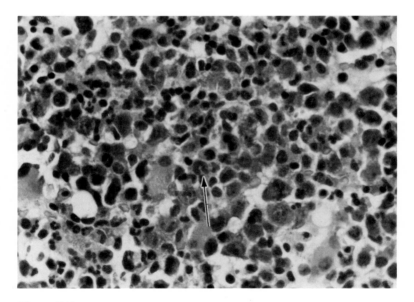

Figure 7-5
Giant band-shaped granulocyte (*arrow*) associated with megaloblastic erythropoiesis. These large, horseshoe-shaped nuclei are easily seen with medium magnification. Compare the giant band-shaped granulocyte with the normal-sized band granulocyte in Figure 7-1. (H&E, ×416.)

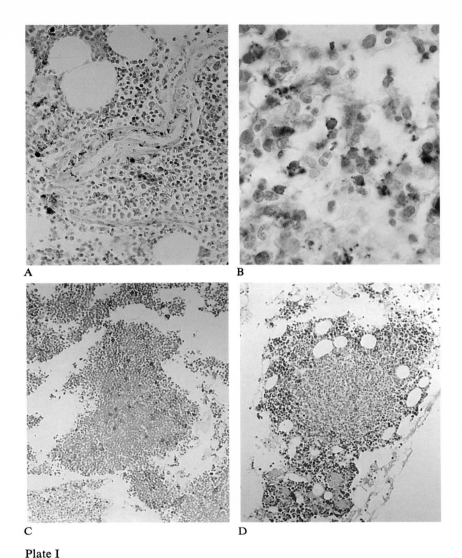

Plate I
(A) Hemosiderin granules in endothelial cells. Ringed sideroblasts are present but cannot be clearly recognized at this magnification. (Gomori's iron reaction, medium power.) (B) Ringed sideroblasts. Note hemosiderin granules surrounding nucleus of normoblast. (Gomori's iron reaction, oil immersion.) (C) Acute myeloblastic leukemia. Absence of fat cells and monotonous appearance of infiltrate. Myelocytes with neutrophilic granules (red) are mixed in with myeloblasts. Compare with D. (Leder, medium power.) (D) Nodule of malignant lymphoma. Myelocytes (red granules) are found only at the periphery of the nodule. Compare with C. (Leder, medium power.)

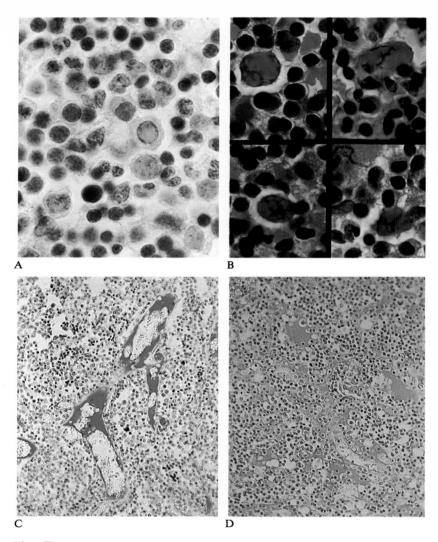

Plate II
(A) Macroglobulinemia. PAS-positive, round intranuclear inclusion (Dutcher body). (PAS, oil immersion.) (B) Macroglobulinemia. Varying appearance of PAS-positive inclusions, apparently intranuclear, compressing chromatin into thin strands. (PAS, oil immersion.) (C) Macroglobulinemia. PAS-positive intravascular plasma in a patient with diffuse lymphocytic infiltration of the marrow. (PAS, medium power.) (D) Macroglobulinemia. PAS-positive, extravascular, lake-like and linear precipitates. (PAS, medium power.) (A, C, and D are reproduced with permission from A. M. Rywlin et al., Bone marrow histology in monoclonal macroglobulinemia. *American Journal of Clinical Pathology* 63:769, 1975.)

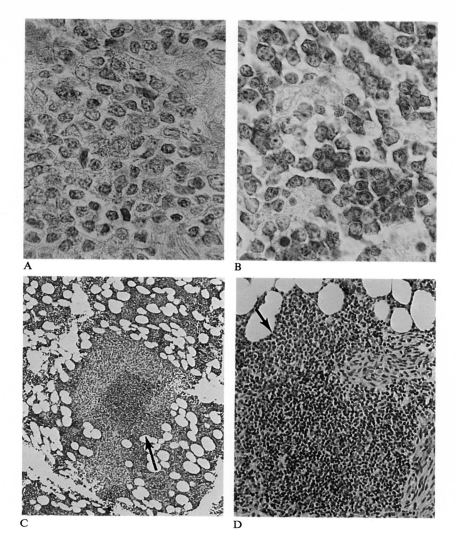

Plate III

(A) Malignant lymphoma, large cell, reticulum cell type (reticulum cell sarcoma, histiocytic lymphoma). Note absence of blue rims of cytoplasm with the Giemsa stain. A few mast cells are also seen. (Giemsa, oil immersion.) (B) Malignant lymphoma, large cell, blast type. Note uniform round to oval nuclei, prominent nucleoli, and dark blue rims of cytoplasm. Compare with A. Also present are a few pale reticulum cells and eosinophils. (Giemsa, oil immersion.) (C) Eosinophilic fibrohistiocytic lesion, type I (lymphofollicular). Mantle of fibrohistiocytes surrounding lymphoid nodule. Dense aggregate of eosinophils is seen at tip of arrow. (H&E, low power.) (D) Higher magnification of lesion shown in C. Central core of lymphocytes, elongated histiocytes, and eosinophils (*arrow*). (H&E, medium power.) (C and D are reproduced from A. M. Rywlin et al., Eosinophilic fibrohistiocytic lesion of bone marrow: A distinctive new morphologic finding, probably related to drug hypersensitivity. *Blood* 40:464–472, 1972. By permission of Grune & Stratton.)

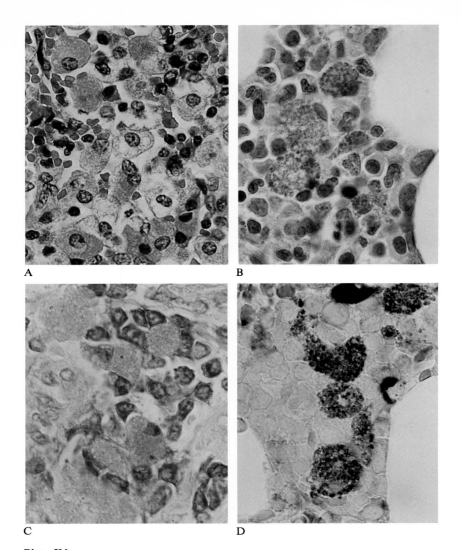

Plate IV
(A) Ceroid (sea-blue) histiocytosis. Note macrophages filled with brown granules and vacuoles. (H&E, oil immersion.) (B) Ceroid (sea-blue) histiocytosis. Ceroid granules (red) are PAS positive. (PAS, oil immersion.) (C) Ceroid (sea-blue) histiocytosis. Ceroid granules stain green-blue with the Giemsa reaction. Note abundant plasma cells. (Giemsa, oil immersion.) (D) Ceroid (sea-blue) histiocytosis. Ceroid granules are Sudan black positive in embedded sections exposed to fat solvents. (Sudan black, oil immersion.) (B, C, and D are reproduced from A. M. Rywlin et al., Ceroid histiocytosis of spleen and bone marrow in idiopathic thrombocytopenic purpura (ITP): A contribution to the understanding of the sea-blue histiocyte. *Blood* 37:587–593, 1971. By permission of Grune & Stratton.)

specific granules. Numerical changes in eosinophilic and basophilic granulocytes are discussed separately. The normal granulocytic series, as seen in histologic sections of in vivo aspirated bone marrow, shows a predominance of segmented neutrophilic granulocytes. Band-shaped granulocytes are next in frequency. Myelocytes are more abundant than promyelocytes, and myeloblasts are inconspicuous.

Granulocytic hyperplasia can occur with a preservation of the ratio of the various maturation stages of the granulocytic series. It can exhibit a "shift to the right," i.e., an increase in the number of segmented granulocytes, or a "shift to the left," an increase in less mature granulocytes. The latter may consist predominantly of band granulocytes, myelocytes, or promyelocytes. A predominantly myeloblastic granulocytic series would more likely represent an acute leukemia than a granulocytic hyperplasia. The distinction between a "reactive"—i.e., nonneoplastic—granulocytic hyperplasia and a leukemia may at times be difficult. This differential diagnosis is discussed under the myeloproliferative disorders.

The term *maturation arrest* has been used to describe a granulocytic series with a predominance of myelocytes and promyelocytes and a sparsity of mature, fully segmented granulocytes (Fig. 7-6). This histologic picture, rather than representing a true maturation arrest, is more likely the result of an increased delivery of more mature granulocytes to the peripheral blood. This results in the depletion of mature granulo-

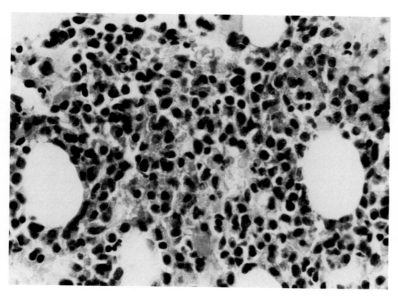

Figure 7-6
"Maturation arrest" of granulocytic series. Note absence of mature polymorphonuclear leukocytes. (H&E, ×416.)

cytes from the bone marrow and a compensatory proliferation of more immature granulocytes.

A true maturation arrest appears to be present in agranulocytosis infantilis hereditaria of Kostmann [6] and in chronic idiopathic neutropenia, in which the bone marrow shows a shift to the left of the granulocytic series with inadequate numbers of fully segmented polymorphonuclear leukocytes.

Granulocytic hyperplasia of the marrow may be due to a variety of causes (see following list).

Causes of Granulocytic Hyperplasia

Infections
Systemic inflammatory diseases (myositis, vasculitis)
Necrosis of tissue (infarcts, necrotic tumor)
Metabolic disorders (uremia, acidosis, eclampsia)
Neoplasms
Hypersplenism
Cortisone therapy (?)
Leukopenia and agranulocytosis caused by drugs and leukoagglutinins
Hereditary infantile agranulocytosis of Kostmann [6]
Preleukemia

It may be associated with normal, increased, or decreased numbers of granulocytes in the circulating pool. Thus leukopenia or agranulocytosis caused by a drug-induced leukoagglutinin is associated with granulocytic hyperplasia. Peripheral blood leukocytosis may be present in the absence of granulocytic hyperplasia of the marrow. This situation, which has been called "pseudoneutrophilia," can be seen under acute stressful conditions when granulocytes are transferred from the marginated pool back to the circulating pool. When patients are treated with cortisone, neutrophilia results from a shift of neutrophils from the marginated to the circulating pool, associated with decreased egress of granulocytes from the circulating blood into tissues and an increased output of granulocytes by the marrow.

A leukemoid reaction is defined as a nonneoplastic leukocytosis exceeding 50,000 cells per cubic milliliter. If the count is less elevated, myelocytes, promyelocytes, and even occasional myeloblasts must be present in the peripheral blood to qualify for a leukemoid reaction. In a leukoerythroblastic reaction, nucleated red blood cells are present in addition to immature granulocytes. Leukemoid reactions, usually neutrophilic, are more rarely eosinophilic, monocytic, or lymphocytic. They may be seen in infectious, toxic, inflammatory, or neoplastic disorders. Leukemoid reactions may occur in patients with carcinomas in the absence of demonstrable bone marrow metastases.

At this time it cannot be resolved whether immature granulocytes and nucleated red blood cells in the peripheral blood are derived from the bone marrow, from foci of extramedullary hematopoiesis, or from both sites.

The bone marrow in leukemoid reactions, as defined above, may have different histologic appearances. There may be myelofibrosis with agnogenic myeloid metaplasia or metastatic carcinoma. The marrow may also show granulocytic hyperplasia with a shift to the right or to the left. In leukemoid reactions marrow fat cells are relatively well preserved and more abundant than in chronic granulocytic leukemia (p. 68). Furthermore, in leukemoid granulocytic reactions the leukocyte alkaline phosphatase is increased, whereas it is decreased in chronic granulocytic leukemia.

Granulocytic Hypoplasia

Granulocytic hypoplasia is defined as an absolute decrease of granulocytic elements in the bone marrow. It implies a decreased M:E ratio caused by a decrease in granulocytes of all stages of maturity. A decrease in the M:E ratio caused by an erythroblastic hyperplasia obviously does not constitute granulocytic hypoplasia. Granulocytic hypoplasia may be due to different causes (see list below). It may be associated with hypoplasia of the red cell and/or megakaryocytic series. Granulocytic hypoplasia is associated with peripheral blood neutropenia. The reverse statement, however, is not necessarily true. Thus "pseudoneutropenia" is caused by a shift of granulocytes from the circulating to the marginated pool without any change in bone marrow granulocytes.

Causes of Granulocytic Hypoplasia

Aplastic anemia
Myelophthisis
Radiation therapy
Drug-induced depression of granulopoiesis
Cyclic neutropenia
Preleukemia

Myeloproliferative Disorders

Under this heading is described the appearance of histologic sections of aspirated bone marrow particles in neoplastic proliferations of the granulocytic series.

Myeloblastic Leukemia

As a rule the bone marrow particles are markedly hypercellular. Only occasional fat cells are found. The discreteness of the individual bone marrow particles is attenuated; they show a tendency to fragmentation and to confluence resulting in sheets of cells. Many of the cells appear to be lying free, unattached to bone marrow particles (Fig. 7-7). Megakaryocytes and nucleated red blood cells are markedly decreased. Cytologically the bone marrow exhibits a monotonous appearance, for it

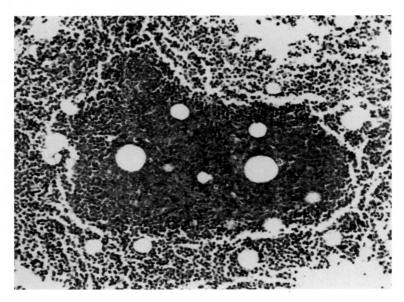

Figure 7-7
Acute myeloblastic leukemia. Note marked decrease in fat cells, monotonous appearance, and attenuation of discreteness of bone marrow particles with many free-lying cells. (H&E, ×130.)

is diffusely infiltrated by cells showing a narrow rim of cytoplasm surrounding round nuclei with prominent nucleoli (Fig. 7-8). These cells cannot be identified with certainty in hematoxylin and eosin-stained sections. A Giemsa stain will bring out a gray-blue rim of cytoplasm and prominent nucleoli, identifying these cells as blasts. A Leder stain will reveal the presence of myelocytes by bringing out their red-stained granules. The myelocytes are sprinkled throughout the sheets of myeloblasts (Plate IC) in contrast to lymphoid infiltrations, in which the myelocytes are decreased and pushed aside to the periphery of the proliferating lymphoid cells (Plate ID). Mature granulocytes are scarce. A study of bone marrow smears helps in the proper identification of the blasts. Reticulin fibers are often slightly increased in myeloblastic leukemia; they seem to be derived from the reticulin fibers that normally surround fat cells.

Occasionally an acute myeloblastic leukemia will present with a hypocellular, predominantly fatty marrow. Clusters of myeloblasts and evidence of poor maturation of the granulocytic series are invariably present. When there is uncertainty whether a marrow represents acute leukemia, it is better to suggest the possibility of a "preleukemic state" and recommend close follow-up studies (p. 73).

In some instances the myeloblastic proliferation may be associated

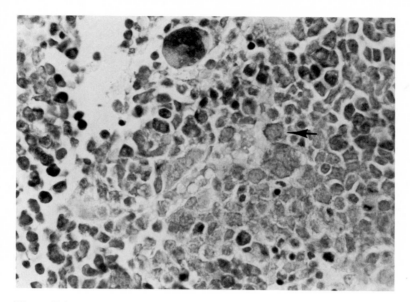

Figure 7-8
Acute myeloblastic leukemia. Monotonous appearance of blasts. Note round
to oval nuclei, prominent nucleoli, and narrow rims of cytoplasm (*arrow*)
which are blue in color. A single megakaryocyte is seen in this field. (Giemsa,
×416.)

with a proliferation of nucleated red cells, which may show megaloblastoid features, as well as a tendency to multinucleation and dyserythropoiesis. These cases may be considered examples of acute erythroleukemia. Even though the diagnosis of acute leukemia is usually easily
made on bone marrow sections, subclassification often requires the
examination of smears and the application of cytochemical and histochemical reactions.

In acute myelomonocytic leukemia the bone marrow contains, in
addition to many characteristic myeloblasts, typical monocytes with
characteristically convoluted nuclei with a loose chromatin structure.
Some of the monocytoid cells contain Leder-positive and peroxidase-
positive granules. The peripheral blood has a more monocytic appearance than the bone marrow, which is obviously myeloblastic.

In acute monocytic leukemia the neoplastic cells resemble mature
monocytes. Immature forms are also seen. Some cases give a positive,
nonspecific esterase reaction. This procedure can be performed on
smears or on unfixed sections of frozen tissue; it cannot be performed on
fixed, Paraplast-embedded tissue.

In acute leukemias, as in other undifferentiated malignant neoplasms,
the neoplastic cells often do not closely resemble known normal

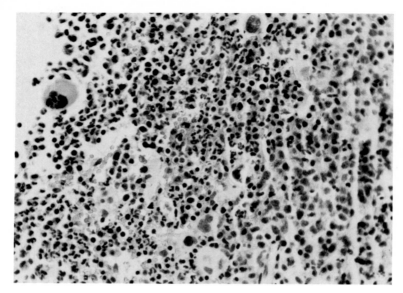

Figure 7-9
Chronic granulocytic leukemia. Hypercellular marrow with increased megakaryocytes associated with many mature and immature granulocytes. In
contrast to polycythemia vera, nucleated red blood cells are relatively inconspicuous. (H&E, ×260.)

counterparts. In such instances, when morphologic appearance and
histochemical markers are inconclusive, we make a diagnosis of undifferentiated acute leukemia.

Most authors consider Ewald's acute leukemic reticuloendotheliosis
to be identical with hairy cell leukemia [see Chap. 9). Some hematologists reserve the term for acute leukemias associated with very large
primitive cells, rather than with the "lymphoid" cells characteristic of
hairy cell leukemia.

Acute Promyelocytic Leukemia

In acute promyelocytic leukemia the bone marrow is overrun by promyelocytes with azurophilic granules. The marked replacement of fat
cells, the decreased megakaryocytes, and the presence of a consumption
coagulopathy aid in the differential diagnosis between a reactive shift to
the left and a promyelocytic leukemia.

Chronic Granulocytic Leukemia

In chronic granulocytic leukemia the bone marrow is markedly hypercellular. Megakaryocytes are increased in number but appear normal
morphologically. The red cell series shows normoblastic maturation.
There is at least a relative decrease in the number of nucleated red blood

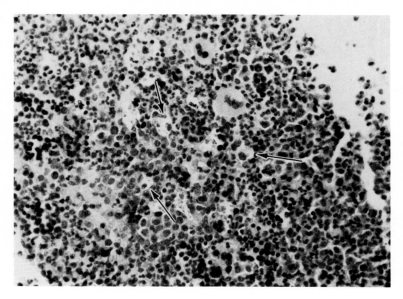

Figure 7-10
Chronic granulocytic leukemia. Empty-appearing spaces (*arrows*), caused by the presence of macrophages, confer to the bone marrow a "starry-sky" appearance (see also Fig. 10-16). (H&E, ×260.)

cells. The granulocytic series is markedly hypercellular and exhibits a normal maturation in the sense that the number of fully segmented polymorphonuclear leukocytes is increased. However, there is also a shift to the left with an increase in the number of myeloblasts, promyelocytes, and myelocytes (Fig. 7-9). There is frequently an increased number of macrophages, giving the particles a starry-sky appearance (Fig. 7-10). Ring-shaped structures made up of platelets with adherent polymorphonuclear leukocytes are often present; Gaucher-like cells may also be seen (see Chap. 10). The increased number of myeloblasts, combined with the increased number of megakaryocytes, the decreased erythroid series, and the decreased leukocyte alkaline phosphatase in the peripheral blood, help to distinguish chronic granulocytic leukemia from a leukemoid reaction. In leukemoid reactions many more fat cells are seen.

In chronic granulocytic leukemia eosinophils are often increased. An increase in basophils can be demonstrated in smears, but these cells cannot be shown in histologic sections of formalin-fixed bone marrow particles because the basophilic granules are water soluble.

Polycythemia Vera

In polycythemia vera the marrow is also markedly hypercellular. Megakaryocytes are increased in number and, contrary to chronic granulo-

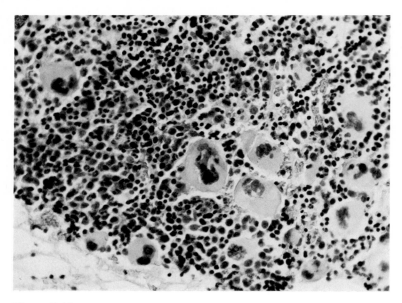

Figure 7-11
Polycythemia vera. Hypercellular marrow with increased number of enlarged megakaryocytes associated with many nucleated red blood cells. (H&E, ×260.)

cytic leukemia, are often enlarged in size and exhibit some nuclear atypism [1]. The red cell series is hypercellular and shows normoblastic maturation (Fig. 7-11). The hemosiderin stores are practically always depleted. The granulocytic series shows normal maturation with an increase in immature forms. Eosinophils are often increased. The number of reticulin fibers is increased and there is a close association between reticulin fibers and megakaryocytes (see Fig. 4-16). We have often observed normal lymphoid nodules in the bone marrow of patients with polycythemia vera.

The combination of an increased number of enlarged megakaryocytes with a prominent hyperplasia of the red cell series is characteristic of polycythemia vera and distinguishes it from chronic granulocytic leukemia, in which the megakaryocytes are associated with many mature granulocytes (see Figs. 7-9, 7-11).

Agnogenic Myeloid Metaplasia
In fully developed agnogenic myeloid metaplasia, bone marrow aspiration is usually unsuccessful. A needle biopsy shows replacement of the fatty marrow with hematopoietic and fibrous tissue. The reticulin fibers are markedly increased, much more so than in chronic granulocytic leukemia or polycythemia vera. Fibroblasts and collagen fibers are also

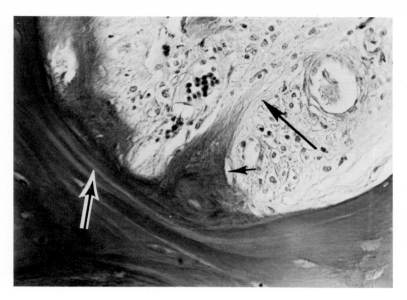

Figure 7-12
Agnogenic myeloid metaplasia. Old lamellar bone (*black-and-white arrow*),
new endosteal bone (*short black arrow*) without parallel lamellae, and fibrosis
of marrow. Note extension of collagen fibers from immature bone into marrow (*long black arrow*). (Van Gieson, ×260.)

prominent, though there are more reticulin than collagen fibers. Megakaryocytes are enlarged and atypical and are often completely surrounded by reticulin fibers. The number of megakaryocytes may be
normal, increased, or decreased. The red cell series is normoblastic and
usually hypocellular. Hemosiderin may be normal, increased, or decreased. The granulocytic series shows normal maturation and may be
numerically increased or decreased. The bone trabeculae may be normal
or show varying degrees of endosteal new bone formation. The new
bone is at first metaplastic (immature bone) and does not show the
regular lamellar appearance of the preexisting trabeculae (Fig. 7-12).
The collagen fibers of the new bone extend into the marrow (Fig.
7-12). The diagnostic features of agnogenic myeloid metaplasia consist
of the increase in reticulin and collagen fibers associated with enlarged
megakaryocytes. The variability of bone marrow histology in agnogenic
myeloid metaplasia is due to the transition stages that exist between
polycythemia vera, chronic granulocytic leukemia, agnogenic myeloid
metaplasia, and acute granulocytic leukemia (Fig 7-13). Polycythemia
vera may evolve into agnogenic myeloid metaplasia. Either of these
conditions may also evolve into chronic granulocytic leukemia. Polycythemia vera, agnogenic myeloid metaplasia, and chronic granulocytic

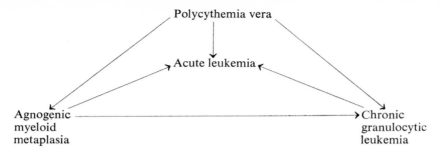

Figure 7-13
Possible transitions between some myeloproliferative disorders.

leukemia may present a "blast crisis," which is essentially an acute blastic leukemia superimposed on the underlying disorder. The evolution from one condition to another is reflected in the bone marrow histology.

Atypical Leukemias

Occasionally the bone marrow does not show all the characteristic findings of a leukemia. This is particularly frequent in elderly patients. It is best in such cases to defer the definitive diagnosis and recommend follow-up studies. Because leukemia is an incurable disease, there is no great urgency in making an early diagnosis. Also, most patients with atypical leukemias do poorly with chemotherapy. Atypical morphologic findings in acute leukemias include increased megakaryocytes, hypocellular marrow, and myelofibrosis. Acute leukemia associated with myelofibrosis and a dry bone marrow tap is discussed under malignant myelosclerosis (see Chap. 11).

Patients with hypocellular marrows in acute leukemia show leukopenia. In the bone marrow islands of myeloblasts are seen. Bone marrow reactions induced by drugs, toxic substances, and radiation therapy may closely mimic an atypical leukemia.

Another atypical leukemia observed in elderly patients is characterized by monocytosis of the peripheral blood associated with islands of myeloblasts and promyelocytes in a focally hypercellular marrow. Otherwise the granulocytic series shows normal maturation. Megakaryocytes appear normal. The red cell series may show some dyserythropoiesis with megaloblastoid features. There may be mild anemia and thrombocytopenia. Miescher and Farquet [4] have called this atypical leukemia "chronic myelomonocytic leukemia of adults." In their series of patients, the 50 percent survival period from the time of diagnosis was 17 months [4]. The differential diagnosis must include tuberculosis, brucellosis, subacute bacterial endocarditis, leishmaniasis, and the recovery phase of agranulocytosis.

In smoldering acute leukemia the patients have symptoms of fatigue or spontaneous bruising for months to years before consulting a physician [5]. The peripheral blood shows mild anemia and moderate thrombocytopenia. The bone marrow may be hypocellular or hypercellular. There is always an increased number of blasts with good preservation of the megakaryocytic and erythroid series.

Preleukemic State

Preleukemic state or syndrome refers to hematologic abnormalities which precede the development of an acute nonlymphocytic leukemia [3]. The incidence of the preleukemic syndrome is unknown. The predominant hematologic abnormality is a refractory anemia that may be associated with thrombocytopenia and neutropenia. Occasional patients exhibit monocytosis or neutrophilia. The peripheral blood smear may show oval macrocytes associated with poikilocytosis and anisocytosis suggestive of B_{12} or folate deficiency. Hypersegmented polymorphonuclear leukocytes, however, are not usually seen. Occasionally hypochromia associated with increased marrow hemosiderin occurs. Dysplastic nucleated red blood cells may also be present in the peripheral smear. Atypical enlarged platelets and hyposegmentation of neutrophils (pseudo-Pelger-Huët anomaly) can be seen. The bone marrow may be hypercellular, hypocellular, or normocellular. Megakaryocytes are usually increased, with somewhat bizarre, hyperchromatic nuclei. The red cell series is often hypercellular and displays megaloblastoid features. Hemosiderin stores are often increased, and ringed sideroblasts may be prominent. The granulocytic series exhibits a slight increase in myeloblasts. Monocytes may be increased.

The preleukemic state may last from a few months to several years. It should be suspected in any refractory anemia, particularly if associated with dyserythropoiesis, ringed sideroblasts, and atypical megakaryocytes.

References

1. Lagerlof, B. Cytophotometric study of megakaryocyte ploidy in polycythemia vera and chronic granulocytic leukemia. *Acta Cytol.* 16:240, 1972.
2. Leder, L. D. Uber die selektive fermentcytochemische Darstellung von neutrophilen myeloischen Zellen und Gewebsmastzellen in Paraffinschnitt. *Klin. Wochenschr.* 43:533, 1964.
3. Linman, J. W., and Saarni, M. I. The preleukemic syndrome. *Semin. Hematol.* 11:93, 1974.
4. Miescher, P. A., and Farquet, J. F. Chronic myelomonocytic leukemia in adults. *Semin. Hematol.* 11:129, 1974.
5. Rheingold, J. F., Kaufman, R., Adelson, E., and Lear, A. Smoldering acute leukemia. *N. Engl. J. Med.* 268:812, 1963.
6. Rohr, K. *Das menschliche Knochenmark.* Stuttgart: Thieme, 1960. P. 283.

8 Plasma Cells, Eosinophils, and Mast Cells

Plasma Cells

Morphology

Plasma cells can be easily identified in histologic sections of aspirated bone marrow particles. They exhibit an eccentrically located, round nucleus surrounded by a discrete basophilic cytoplasm. The nucleus often shows a characteristic appearance: coarse clumps of chromatin are located close to the nuclear membrane and are separated from each other by lighter parachromatin. This appearance has been likened to the spokes of a wheel. A paranuclear halo corresponding to the Golgi apparatus is often present (Fig. 8-1). When plasma cells are increased in number, a few contain two or more nuclei. The cytoplasm of the plasma cells may display round or oval eosinophilic inclusions of varying sizes called Russell bodies (Fig. 8-2). Though these inclusions are uniformly eosinophilic their reactions with the Giemsa stain vary. This variable appearance of Russell bodies with the Giemsa stain has given rise to different names: Mott cell, grape cell, and morular cell. These cytoplasmic inclusions may be PAS positive or negative. Occasionally plasma cells contain eosinophilic, PAS positive, intranuclear inclusions (Dutcher bodies) (Plate IIA) that may represent intracytoplasmic inclusions which have invaginated the nuclear membrane and therefore appear to be intranuclear in position with light microscopy. According to Brittin et al. [5] these inclusions are true nuclear bodies and represent nuclear elaboration of glycoprotein. Maldonado et al. [23] concluded on the basis of light and electron microscopic studies that Russell bodies and intranuclear inclusions are morphologically identical. They suggested that the intranuclear bodies represent true intranuclear inclusions which are probably of cytoplasmic origin. In my bone marrow collection Russell bodies are more frequently found in nonneoplastic plasma cells, whereas intranuclear inclusions are more frequent in macroglobulinemia, lymphoma, and myeloma. We have observed peculiar eosinophilic, PAS-positive inclusions in patients with macroglobulinemia (monoclonal or polyclonal) as well as in myeloma and malignant lymphoma associated with IgA monoclonal gammopathy. These inclusions, which occupy the entire cell, are angular and are separated from each other by what appear to be strands of chromatin (Fig. 8-3, Plate IIB). A complete nucleus cannot be recognized in these cells. It is unlikely that these cells represent histologic sections of Waldenström's thesaurocytes [34], cells which are clearly recognizable in smears and which contain a distinct nucleus and cytoplasmic inclusions. Plasma

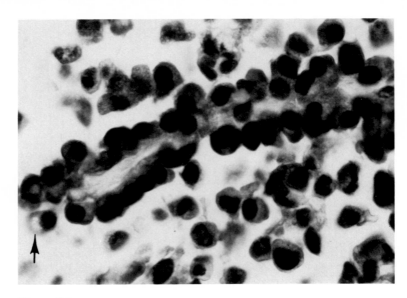

Figure 8-1
Typical appearance of plasma cell in histologic sections: eccentric, round,
dark nucleus with distinct paranuclear halo (*arrow*). Note perivascular clus-
tering. (H&E, ×1100.)

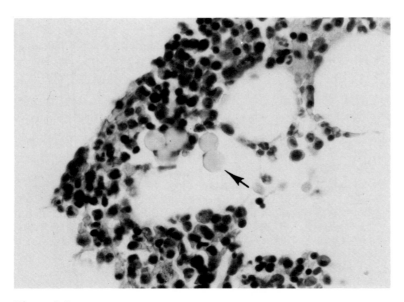

Figure 8-2
Characteristic appearance of Russell bodies (*arrow*): round, hyaline droplets.
(H&E, ×504.)

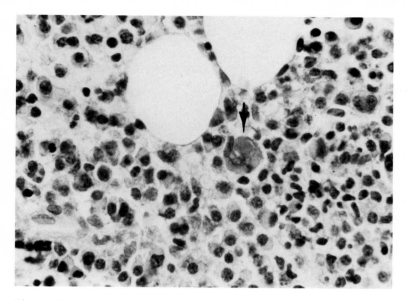

Figure 8-3
Eosinophilic, somewhat angular cellular inclusions separated by strands of chromatin (*arrow*) (see also Plate IIB). (H&E, ×556.)

cells may also contain varyingly shaped crystalline inclusions. The recognition of "flaming" plasma cells has not been accomplished with certainty in tissue sections. In smears, flaming plasma cells exhibit a red hue of their peripheral cytoplasm.

Distribution

In normal marrow plasma cells characteristically surround small blood vessels in a single layer (Fig. 8-4). In reactive plasmacytosis of the bone marrow the perivascular plasmacellular cuff may be two or three layers thick. Plasma cells are also seen at the edge of lymphoid nodules and occasionally mixed with other hematopoietic cells. Lipid granulomas invariably contain a few plasma cells (see Chap. 11).

Numerical Considerations

No exact numerical data are available as to normal numbers of plasma cells in histologic sections of bone marrow. In normal bone marrow it is rare to find clumps containing more than 4 or 5 plasma cells. In bone marrow smears most authors consider 2 to 3 percent as the upper limit of normal for plasma cells.

In hypogammaglobulinemia and agammaglobulinemia, plasma cells are markedly decreased or absent. Plasma cells may be considerably increased in many conditions (see list on p. 78).

Conditions Associated with Nonneoplastic Bone Marrow Plasmacytosis
(Bone marrow plasmacytosis is a constant finding in some of these conditions, variable in others.)

Chronic infections, pneumonia, tuberculosis, typhoid fever, lymphopathia venereum, chronic pyelonephritis
Kala azar
Drug reactions, agranulocytosis
Collagen diseases, lupus erythematosus, rheumatoid arthritis
Periarteritis nodosa
Sarcoidosis [9]
Allergic reactions, serum sickness
Cirrhosis of the liver
Metastatic carcinoma
Hodgkin's disease
Gaucher's disease
Ceroid histiocytosis (sea-blue histiocytosis) [31]
Pregnancy
Polyclonal gammopathy
Benign monoclonal gammopathy
Anemia, particularly iron deficiency anemia
Diabetes mellitus
Primary amyloidosis

In general, bone marrow plasmacytosis is seen in diseases associated with hypergammaglobulinemia. Also, there appears to be a fair correlation between numbers of bone marrow plasma cells and the degree of hypergammaglobulinemia. The presence of increased numbers of plasma cells in association with increased numbers of histiocytes such as seen in Gaucher's disease or with ceroid histiocytosis [31] is more difficult to explain. Perhaps the increase in plasma cells in these conditions is related to their tendency, even in normal marrows, to cluster around a histiocyte, a phenomenon first described by Rohr [30], called plasmacytic satellitosis, and studied extensively by Hyun et al. [16]. These authors found plasmacytic satellitosis in 10 percent of bone marrows without plasmacytosis and in 46.4 percent of marrows with plasmacytosis. Plasmacytic satellitosis was not observed in myeloma [16].

Myeloma
The essential pathologic process in myeloma is a neoplastic proliferation of plasma cells in the bone marrow associated with characteristic electrophoretic and immunoelectrophoretic patterns in serum and/or urine. Diffuse osteopenia and/or punched-out osteolytic lesions are usually present when the disease is fully developed. A diagnosis of multiple myeloma must be based on the demonstration of a neoplastic proliferation of plasma cells in the bone marrow. When the disease is fully developed, the diagnosis is easily made by finding in bone marrow smears or sections extensive replacement of the normal fatty and

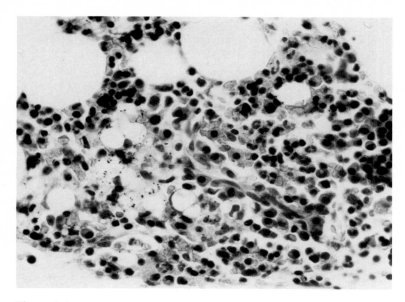

Figure 8-4
Perivascular plasma cells in reactive (inflammatory) plasmacytosis. Note elongated endothelial cell nuclei with adjacent plasma cells and lipid granuloma with finely granular black pigment (see also Fig. 11-19). (H&E, ×416.)

hematopoietic marrow by sheets of plasma cells. Bone marrow aspirations are often performed because of monoclonal gammopathies found in oligosymptomatic patients. In such cases a differential diagnosis between an inflammatory and a neoplastic plasmacytosis may be difficult.

The differentiation between a neoplastic and nonneoplastic proliferation of plasma cells can be made more reliably in histologic sections than in smears of the bone marrow [6]. The criteria used on smears are mainly numerical and cytologic. The numerical criterion is arbitrary; if plasma cells exceed 20 to 30 percent, the plasmacytosis is presumably myelomatous. The cytologic criteria include the presence of large, young, and abnormal plasma cells. The plasma cells may be multinucleated, and the nuclei often contain large nucleoli whose diameter is equal to or exceeds one-third of the diameter of the nucleus. These criteria are useful, but they are not as reliable as histologic criteria because myelomatous cells may not be distinguishable cytologically from reactive plasma cells.

The most helpful histologic finding in the distinction between inflammatory and myelomatous plasmacytosis is the presence of solid collections of plasma cells. "Solid" refers to the absence of fat cells (Fig. 8-5). These solid collections of plasma cells are less conspicuous under low magnification than lymphoid nodules, because plasma cells are less tightly aggregated than lymphocytes, and plasmacytic collections are less

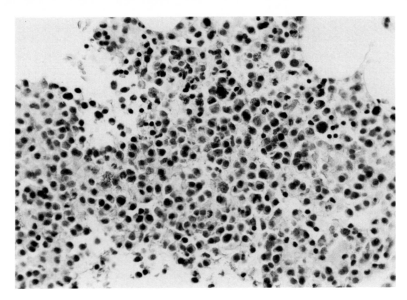

Figure 8-5
Solid (absence of fat cells) aggregate of plasma cells in a case of myeloma. Note replacement of fat cells, and poor differentiation and variability of plasma cells. (H&E, ×296.)

discrete than lymphoid nodules. Indeed around the periphery of the solid collection of plasma cells one observes variable infiltration of plasma cells into the septa between fat cells (Fig. 8-6). In my experience solid collections of plasma cells are diagnostic of myeloma if they measure at least 0.2 mm in greatest dimension. This corresponds approximately to half a high dry power field using an AO microscope with 10 × oculars and a 40 × objective. It is this replacement of fat cells and hematopoietic elements which is characteristic of neoplastic plasmacytosis. A reticulin stain often reveals an increased number of fibers in such solid collections (Fig. 8-7). These fibers presumably are the remnants of the reticulin fibers which surround normal fat cells.

Such solid plasmacytic collections may be present in only one or two of many aspirated particles. The remaining particles may be normocellular or hypocellular (Fig. 8-8). In such cases a diagnosis of myeloma can be missed if only smears are examined.

In more advanced cases of myeloma the entire bone marrow particle may be replaced by sheets of plasma cells. In such cases there is often hemorrhage into the solid collections of plasma cells. Occasionally these collections are associated with an increased number of eosinophils or mast cells (Fig. 8-9).

Another histologic criterion for the diagnosis of myeloma is the plasma cell infiltrate. Here the fat cells are preserved or slightly de-

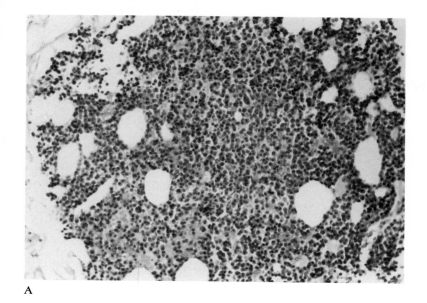

A

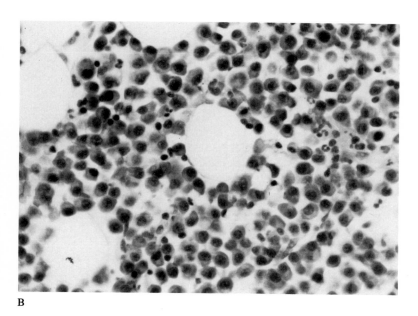

B

Figure 8-6
(A) Multiple myeloma. Solid collections of plasma cells (*center*) and infiltration of plasma cells into septa separating fat cells. At this magnification the plasma cells are difficult to recognize. (H&E, ×130.) (B) Higher magnification of A. Note a few polymorphonuclear leukocytes admixed with plasma cells. (H&E, ×570.)

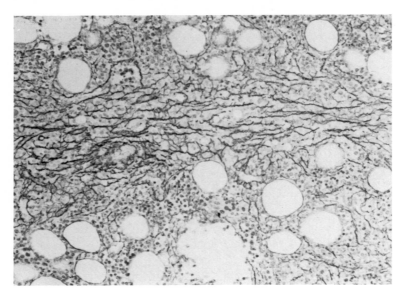

Figure 8-7
Accentuated reticulin framework in a case of IgA myeloma. (Gordon-Sweets',
×160.)

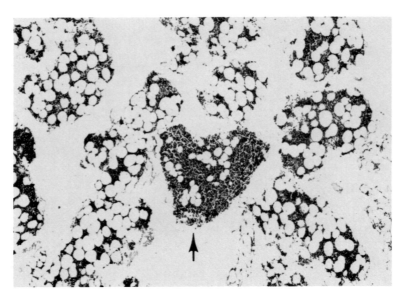

Figure 8-8
Multiple myeloma. Only one of the aspirated particles is involved (*arrow*).
The other particles are normocellular. (H&E, ×48.)

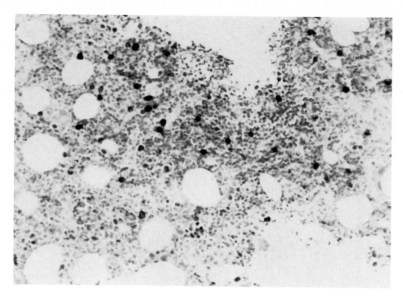

Figure 8-9
Increased number of mast cells in a case of multiple myeloma. At this magnification the plasma cells in the solid area cannot be recognized. The mast
cells appear as dark dots. (Giemsa, ×150.)

creased and the plasma cells are present in the septa separating individual fat cells. This can be called an interstitial infiltrate. The septa
separating the fat cells may contain a single layer of plasma cells or
more frequently are broadened by several layers of plasma cells (Fig.
8-10). A few hematopoietic cells may be seen among the plasma cells.
This plasmacytic infiltrate is usually seen at the margin of solid collections. If plasmacytic infiltrates are present without solid plasmacytic
collections, the diagnosis of a myelomatous process is less certain, particularly if such infiltrates are seen only in an occasional bone marrow
particle. It is best in such instances to repeat the marrow aspiration and
search for the presence of solid plasmacytic collections. A perivascular
distribution of plasma cells, though by far more frequent in reactive
plasmacytosis, can also be seen in myeloma (Fig. 8-11). The presence
of many immature cells sometimes resembling reticulum cells speaks in
favor of myeloma. Intranuclear and intracytoplasmic inclusions can be
seen in both neoplastic and nonneoplastic plasmacytosis. Among the
neoplastic processes, intranuclear inclusions are most frequent in macroglobulinemia and in lymphoma or myeloma associated with an IgA
peak.

Light-chain myeloma can often be suspected morphologically when
the myeloma cells are very uniform and look like mature plasma cells or
plasmacytoid lymphocytes. Inside the solid collections the cells appear

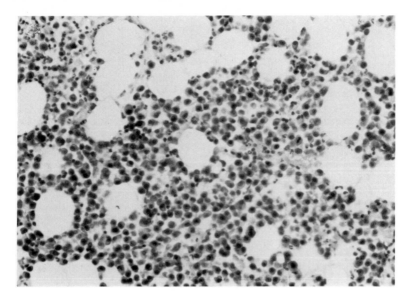

Figure 8-10
Light chain myeloma. Plasmacytic infiltrate with relative preservation of fat cells. (H&E, ×200.)

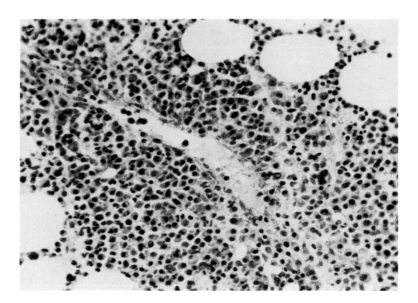

Figure 8-11
IgA myeloma. Perivascular sheets of plasma cells. In inflammatory plasmacytosis only two or three layers of plasma cells are seen around blood vessels. (H&E, ×267.)

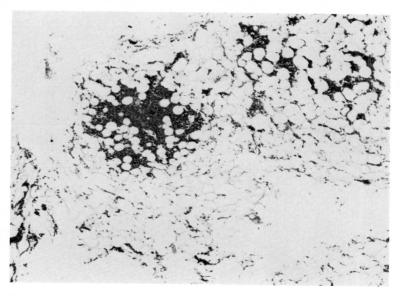

Figure 8-12
Treated multiple myeloma. Focus of myeloma in hypocellular marrow.
Plasma cells cannot be recognized at this magnification. (H&E, ×55.)

to have a somewhat linear arrangement. The reticulin framework is
moderately increased.

In treated multiple myeloma the bone marrow particles are often
hypocellular and only an occasional particle will show a solid collection
or an infiltrate of plasma cells (Fig. 8-12). The hypocellular particles
often display fibrinous myelitis, which is characteristic of chemotherapy
and radiation therapy (see Figs. 11-14, 11-15). Occasionally hyaline
scars are seen following chemotherapy or radiotherapy. These scars
replace partially solid collections of myeloma cells (Fig. 8-13). Such
scars have to be differentiated from amyloidosis and paramyloidosis.
With the van Gieson stain they have the characteristic red color of
collagen. They stain reddish with Congo red but fail to show the typical
dichroism of amyloid deposits. We diagnose amyloidosis when we can
demonstrate Congo-red positivity with dichroism, fluorescence with
thioflavine, and metachromasia with crystal violet. We use the term
paramyloidosis in its original sense, for hyaline deposits which give one
or two, but not all, of the characteristic reactions of amyloid.

We have observed solid collections of plasma cells located centrally
within lymphoid nodules in a 70-year-old man with diffuse lung disease
of unknown etiology and monoclonal IgG gammopathy (Fig. 8-14).
This constitutes a unique observation in our material. In some areas
there were more than 4 lymphoid nodules per low power field. Our

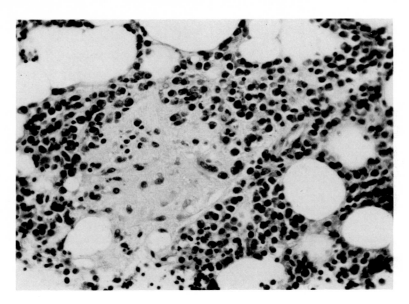

Figure 8-13
Multiple myeloma treated with radiotherapy. Hyaline scar partially replaces solid collection of plasma cells. (H&E, ×267.)

presumptive diagnosis was lymphoproliferative disorder (probably malignant lymphoma) with plasma cell differentiation.

Benign Monoclonal Gammopathy

All patients with monoclonal gammopathies should have a bone marrow examination. The bone marrow of patients with benign monoclonal gammopathy exhibits normal or moderately increased numbers of plasma cells. Solid collections of plasma cells or plasma cell infiltrates are not found. Because the involvement of the bone marrow in myeloma may be spotty, it is obvious that one negative bone marrow aspiration does not rule out myeloma. If the electrophoretic data suggest a benign monoclonal gammopathy, and a single bone marrow examination fails to reveal myeloma, the diagnosis of benign monoclonal gammopathy is accepted and the patient is restudied in 6 months. Electrophoretic data suggesting a benign monoclonal gammopathy include a modest elevation of the monoclonal immunoglobulin, no significant depression of the other immunoglobulins, a normal serum albumin, and the absence of light chains in the urine. If, on the other hand, electrophoretic data suggest a myeloma and a first marrow aspirate fails to reveal myelomatous nodules or infiltrates, repeat marrows at different sites are performed.

Macroglobulinemia is discussed in Chapter 9.

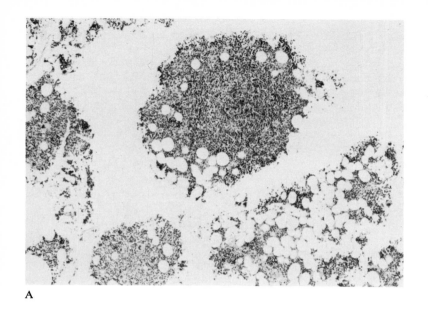

A

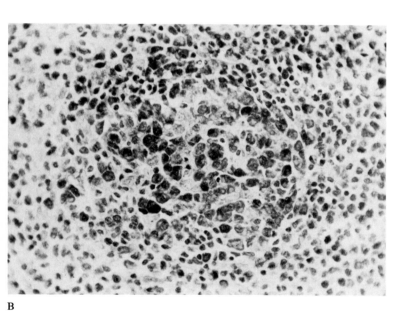

B

Figure 8-14
(A) Lymphoproliferative disorder with nodules of lymphocytes with centrally located plasma cells (see B). (H&E, ×58.) (B) Higher power of A showing plasma cells in the center of the lymphoid nodule. (Giemsa, ×307.)

Heavy-Chain Disease

It appears from the literature that in gamma heavy-chain disease the marrow may be normal [7] or may show erythroid [19] or myeloid [11] hyperplasia. It may exhibit increased numbers of plasma cells [33] or lymphocytes at various stages of development with an admixture of plasma cells, reticulum cells, and eosinophils [4, 18, 27].

In mu-chain disease the marrow resembles chronic lymphocytic leukemia but also contains vacuolated plasma cells [20].

In alpha heavy-chain disease the bone marrow may be normal or may exhibit an increase in plasma cells [35].

Eosinophils

Morphology

Eosinophilic leukocytes are easily recognized in hematoxylin and eosin-stained histologic sections. Their hallmark is the eosinophilic granule, which is larger and more distinct than the neutrophilic granule and which is rich in peroxidase. On electron microscopy the eosinophilic granules display a crystalloid core. The Charcot-Leyden crystals, which form when large numbers of eosinophils disintegrate and liberate their granules, are probably derived from these crystalloid cores.

Eosinophils are attracted by "allergic" events. There is some evidence that eosinophils elaborate plasminogen and are attracted by fibrin deposits [28, 29].

Eosinophilic myelocytes have a round, somewhat eccentric nucleus, which is smaller than the nucleus of neutrophilic myelocytes. In smears a few basophilic granules may be seen among the eosinophilic ones. The eosinophilic metamyelocyte shows an indented nucleus. The fully segmented eosinophilic leukocyte exhibits, as a rule, only two lobes. Multilobed eosinophils are relatively rare.

Numerical Considerations

Eosinophils are found in the bone marrow associated with other cells of the granulocytic series. They are increased in the immediate vicinity of lymphoid nodules. A marked increase in eosinophils can be easily recognized in tissue sections of bone marrow particles. Minor increases are less readily diagnosed because of inadequate data about normal numbers of eosinophils in histologic sections. This problem is further complicated by the considerable variability in the number of eosinophils in different marrow particles. A definite increase in eosinophils may also be spotty. It is generally accepted that about 4 percent of the cells in bone marrow smears are eosinophils [30].

Dissociations between peripheral blood, tissue, and bone marrow eosinophil content have been frequently noted. In part such dissociations may be explained by temporal factors. Chemotactic attraction of eosinophils by a target tissue, such as the lung or appendix, may cause a temporary disappearance of eosinophils from the peripheral blood. This in turn causes a transfer of eosinophils from the bone marrow to the peripheral blood, causing a temporary decrease in bone marrow eosinophils.

Absence of bone marrow eosinophils has been reported in patients who have agammaglobulinemia with thymoma [14] and in a patient with bronchial asthma [12]. Absence of eosinophils from the bone marrow, peripheral blood, and nasal secretions has been reported in a patient with kappa-chain deficiency [3].

The disappearance of eosinophils from the peripheral blood, as seen in infectious diseases such as typhoid fever or following the administration of corticosteroids, is not associated with disappearance of eosinophils from the bone marrow. In some leukemoid reactions bone marrow eosinophils may be increased.

Bone marrow eosinophilia may be associated with different conditions (see following list).

Conditions Associated with Bone Marrow Eosinophilia
(The increased number of eosinophils is a constant finding in some of these conditions, variable in others.)

Allergic reactions: focal eosinophilia; diffuse eosinophilia; eosinophilic fibrohistiocytic lesion (see Chap. 11); granulomatous inflammation with eosinophilia (see Chap. 11)
Parasitic infestation
Skin diseases
Carcinoma: metastatic carcinoma to bone marrow; eosinophilia without evidence of bone marrow carcinoma
Hodgkin's disease: Hodgkin's disease of bone marrow; eosinophilia without evidence of bone marrow involvement
Myeloma
Eosinophilic granuloma
Periarteritis nodosa
Hematologic conditions: chronic myeloproliferative diseases; eosinophilic leukemia
Familial eosinophilia [32]
Familial reticuloendotheliosis with eosinophilia [26]
Hypereosinophilic diseases [8]: eosinophilic pneumonitis, endocarditis, gastroenteritis, prostatitis, collagen disease [25]
Eosinophilic leukemia

Two drug-related bone marrow lesions associated with increased eosinophils are described in Chapter 11. In the eosinophilic fibrohistiocytic lesions we have seen eosinophilic microabscesses associated with a fibrohistiocytic proliferation in relation to lymphoid follicles (Chap. 11; Plate IIIC, D). The drug-related granulomatous inflammation of the bone marrow shows a rather diffuse proliferation of histiocytes associated with a sprinkling of eosinophils (Chap. 11).

I have not had the occasion to study tissue sections of aspirated marrow in eosinophilic leukemia. In a smear the differentiation between a reactive and a neoplastic eosinophilic proliferation may be quite difficult, and one has to rely on cytologic criteria of size and immaturity of eosinophils as well as the associated finding of increased numbers of myeloblasts [2]. An eosinophilic leukemoid reaction preceding a myeloblastic leukemia has to be considered in the differential diagnosis of eosinophilic leukemia. Judging from autopsy findings, one would expect the criteria for the diagnosis of eosinophilic leukemia to be similar to those for myeloma, that is, significant solid replacement of fatty and hematopoietic marrow by aggregates of eosinophils [30]. How large a "significant" solid aggregate of eosinophils has to be before a diagnosis of eosinophilic leukemia is justified cannot be stated at the present time.

In recent years the term *hypereosinophilic syndrome* has been introduced to describe a spectrum of diseases characterized by persistent eosinophilia of the blood and organ infiltration by eosinophils [8]. Eosinophilic leukemia is viewed as one pole of the spectrum. The hypereosinophilic syndrome includes such entities as disseminated eosinophilic collagen disease and Löffler's fibroplastic endocarditis. Eosinophilia of the marrow is often present in these cases. It is not established that the "lumping" of different disease entities characterized by eosinophilia is justified.

The bone marrow eosinophilia associated with many of the conditions given in the preceding list is not obligatory. Eosinophilia may be present in all the aspirated bone marrow particles or in only some of them. The involvement of each particle may be spotty or diffuse.

Mast Cells

Morphology

Mast cells are rather difficult to recognize in hematoxylin and eosin-stained sections of bone marrow particles. However, they can be recognized easily with the Giemsa, Leder, and PAS stains (see Appendix, 1, 5, 7). With the Giemsa stain the mast cells reveal a diffuse distribution of granules often obscuring the nucleus and the cellular outline. The nuclei of the mast cells are much better seen with the PAS stain. They appear rather small, round to oval, and eccentric. The cytoplasm of mast cells is PAS positive but only faintly granular. With the PAS stain the mast cell appears round to oval and occasionally more elongated. According to Lennert [22], only two-thirds of the mast cells are PAS positive. With the Leder stain the mast cell granules appear bright red. Mast cell granules can also be stained with toluidine blue and Bismarck brown.

Basophilic Leukocytes

Basophilic leukocytes cannot be demonstrated in tissue sections of formalin-fixed bone marrow particles, because the basophilic granules are water soluble [21]. There is disagreement in the literature as to the solubility of the granules of basophilic leukocytes in absolute alcohol [17, 21]. I have not attempted to demonstrate basophilic leukocytes in bone marrow particles fixed in absolute alcohol.

Distribution and Function

In tissue sections mast cells are seen in close relationship to blood vessels and lymphoid nodules. Some mast cells are seen in foci of granulocytopoiesis. The distribution of mast cells may be spotty and varies from particle to particle. In bone marrow biopsies mast cells are often most numerous in the proximity of bone trabeculae. In bone marrow smears the mast cells are most abundant in the thick areas of crushed particles. Mast cells viewed with the Giemsa stain have to be distinguished from ceroid-containing histiocytes (sea-blue histiocytes, see Chap. 10), hemosiderin-containing histiocytes, melanophages, and melanocytes. Ceroid-containing histiocytes are not as densely granulated as mast cells, and the nucleus is clearly visible. In hematoxylin and eosin-stained sections, ceroid has a brownish hue. Hemosiderin displays with the Giemsa stain a greenish blue hue, rather than the dark blue color of mast cell granules or the navy blue tint of ceroid. Also, hemosiderin granules vary considerably in size and can be easily seen in hematoxylin and eosin-stained sections, whereas mast cell granules do not stain with hematoxylin and eosin. With the Giemsa stain, melanin has a bluish green appearance which is different from mast cells. Melanocytes in the bone marrow have neoplastic appearing nuclei with prominent nucleoli, quite different from the bland histiocytic nuclei of melanophages. If the pigment obscures the nuclei, the tissue has to be bleached to distinguish melanophages from melanocytes.

Mast cell granules contain nonsulfated and sulfated acid mucopolysaccharides: hyaluronic acid, heparin, and chondroitin sulfates. Mast cells synthesize histamine. Serotonin has been demonstrated in the mast cells of the mouse and rat. There is no conclusive evidence that serotonin exists in human mast cells.

Mast cells are indirectly involved in the formation of fibrous tissue [1]. An immediate tissue response to edema is degranulation of mast cells. The water is bound by the liberated mucopolysaccharides and is transformed into a hydrated gel constituting the mucinous ground substance. The mere presence of acid mucopolysaccharides seems to stimulate the production of collagen [1].

Adrenocortical steroids with glucocorticoid effects reduce the number of identifiable mast cells [1]. Administration of such steroids results in a decreased content of acid mucopolysaccharides in the ground substance. Thyrotropic hormone, on the other hand, seems to stimulate the synthetic activity of mast cells. This effect is counteracted by thyroid hormone.

Numerical Considerations

Inadequate data are available on normal numbers of mast cells in tissue sections of aspirated bone marrow. A systematic study on the appearance and significance of mast cells in human bone marrow was reported by Johnstone [17], who stressed the advantage of sections over smears in the evaluation of mast cells. No mast cells were seen in 30 percent of the patients. A few mast cells were found in 60 percent, and 10 percent of the patients exhibited abundant mast cells. The presence or numbers of mast cells bore no relation to the iron content or degree of erythropoiesis of the marrow. No single factor could be correlated with the increase of mast cells [17]. Conditions in which we have found increased numbers of mast cells are listed below. In some of these conditions, the increased number of mast cells has not been a consistent feature. Increased numbers of mast cells may be associated with increased eosinophils and plasma cells.

Conditions Associated with Increased Number of Mast Cells in the Bone Marrow
(The increased number of mast cells is a constant finding in some of these conditions, variable in others.)

Systemic mastocytosis
Mast cell leukemia
Refractory anemias
Lymphoproliferative disorders with macroglobulinemia
Nodular lymphoid hyperplasia of bone marrow (see Chap. 9)
Myeloma
Metastatic carcinoma
Atrophy of bone marrow (after irradiation or chemotherapy)
Myelofibrosis
Osteoporosis [13]
Uremia with dialysis [24]

In systemic mastocytosis the characteristic findings consist of skin lesions, hepatosplenomegaly, and lymphadenopathy. Rarely mastocytosis can occur without cutaneous manifestations. Occasionally in a patient with hepatosplenomegaly an increased number of mast cells in the bone marrow may be the first clue that systemic mastocytosis is the underlying disease [15]. A leukemic picture may occur in the course of systemic mastocytosis [10]. The marrow in mastocytosis may exhibit fibrosis; the bone may show focal or diffuse resorption or new bone formation.

References

1. Asboe-Hansen, G.   Mast cells in health and disease. *Bull. N.Y. Acad. Sci.* 44:1048, 1968.
2. Benvenisti, D. S., and Ulfmann, J. E.   Eosinophilic leukemia: Report of five cases and review of the literature. *Ann. Intern. Med.* 71:731, 1969.
3. Bernier, G. M., Gunderman, J. R., and Ruymann, F. B.   Kappa-chain deficiency. *Blood* 40:795, 1972.

4. Bloch, K. J., Lee, L., Mills, J. A., and Haber, E.   Gamma heavy chain disease: An expanding clinical and laboratory spectrum. *Am. J. Med.* 55:61, 1973.
5. Brittin, G. M., Tanaka, Y., and Brecher, G.   Intranuclear inclusions in multiple myeloma and macroglobulinemia. *Blood* 21:335, 1963.
6. Canale, D. D., and Collins, R. D.   Use of bone marrow particle sections in the diagnosis of multiple myeloma. *Am. J. Clin. Pathol.* 61:382, 1974.
7. Case records of the Massachusetts General Hospital. *N. Engl. J. Med.* 282:1332, 1970.
8. Chusid, M. J., Dale, D. C., West, B. C., and Wolff, S. M.   The hypereosinophilic syndrome: Analysis of fourteen cases with review of the literature. *Medicine* (Balt.) 54:1, 1975.
9. Cohen, S., and Civantos, F.   Sarcoidosis with plasmacytosis. *J.A.M.A.* 205:250, 1968.
10. Efrati, P., Klajman, A., and Spitz, H.   Mast cell leukemia? Malignant mastocytosis with leukemia-like manifestations. *Blood* 2:869, 1957.
11. Ellman, L. L., and Bloch, K. J.   Heavy chain disease: Report of a seventh case. *N. Engl. J. Med.* 278:1195, 1968.
12. Forssman, O., and Korgren, M.   Aneosinophilia in a patient with bronchial asthma. *Acta Med. Scand.* 172:1, 1962.
13. Frame, B., and Nixon, R. K.   Bone-marrow mast cells in osteoporosis of aging. *N. Engl. J. Med.* 279:626, 1968.
14. Gatti, R. A., and Good, R. A.   Lymphoreticular Disorders—Benign Abnormalities of Immunoglobulin Synthesis. In W. J. Williams, E. Beutler, A. J. Erslev, and R. W. Rundles (Eds.), *Hematology*. New York: McGraw-Hill, 1972. P. 863.
15. Gonella, J. S., and Lipsey, A. I.   Mastocytosis manifested by hepatosplenomegaly. *N. Engl. J. Med.* 271:533, 1964.
16. Hyun, B. H., Kwa, D., Gabaldon, H., and Ashton, J. K.   Reactive plasmacytic lesions of the bone marrow. *Am. J. Clin. Pathol.* 65:921, 1976.
17. Johnstone, J. M.   The appearance and significance of tissue mast cells in human bone marrow. *J. Clin. Pathol.* 7:275, 1954.
18. Keller, H., Spengler, G. A., Skvanil, F., Flury, W., Noseda, G., and Riva, G.   Zur Frage der heavy chain disease. *Schweiz. Med. Wochenschr.* 100:1012, 1970.
19. Lebreton, J. P., Rivat, C., Rivat, L., Guillemot, L., and Ropartz, C.   La maladie des chaînes lourdes. *Presse Med.* 75:2251, 1967.
20. Lee, S. L., Rosner, F., Ruberman, W., and Glasberg, S.   Mu-chain disease. *Ann. Intern. Med.* 75:407, 1971.
21. Lennert, K.   Zur Praxis der pathologisch-anatomischen Knochenmarksuntersuchung. *Frankf. Z. Pathol.* 63:267, 1952.
22. Lennert, K.   Lymphknoten. In O. Lubarsch, F. Henke, R. Roessle, and E. Uehlinger (Eds.), *Handbuch der speziellen pathologischen Anatomie und Histologie*. Berlin: Springer, 1961. Vol. I, pt. 3, pp. 104–120.
23. Maldonado, J. E., Brown, A. L., Bayrd, E. D., and Pease, G. L.   Cytoplasmic and intranuclear electron-dense bodies in the myeloma cell. *Arch. Pathol.* 81:484, 1966.
24. Neiman, R. S., Bischel, M. D., and Lukes, R. J.   Uremia and mast cell proliferation. *Lancet* 1:959, 1972.
25. Odeberg, B.   Eosinophilic leukemia and disseminated eosinophilic collagen disease. *Acta Med. Scand.* 177:129, 1965.

26. Omenn, G. S.   Familial reticuloendotheliosis with eosinophilia. *N. Engl. J. Med.* 273:427, 1965.
27. Osserman, E. F., and Takatsuki, K.   Clinical and immunochemical studies of four cases of heavy (Hgamma²) chain disease. *Am. J. Med.* 37:351, 1964.
28. Rebuck, J. W., Sweet, L. O., and Barth, C. L.   Increased fibrin deposition in allergic inflammation in relation to eosinophil migrations. *Fed. Proc.* 26:745, 1967.
29. Riddle, J. M., and Barnhart, M. I.   The eosinophil as a source for profibrinolysin in acute inflammation. *Blood* 25:776, 1965.
30. Rohr, K.   *Das menschliche Knochenmark.* Stuttgart: Thieme, 1960. Pp. 315, 349.
31. Rywlin, A. M., Lopez-Gomez, A., Tachmes, P., and Pardo, V.   Ceroid histiocytosis of the spleen in hyperlipemia: Relationship to the syndrome of the sea-blue histiocyte. *Am. J. Clin. Pathol.* 56:572, 1971.
32. Stefanini, M., and Kavara, M.   Familial eosinophilia and splenomegaly. *Am. J. Med. Sci.* 245:125, 1963.
33. Tsuji, T.   Heavy chain (Fc fragment) disease. *Acta Haematol. Jap.* 33:89, 1970.
34. Waldenström, J.   *Diagnosis and Treatment of Multiple Myeloma.* New York: Grune & Stratton, 1970. P. 20.
35. Zlotnick, A., and Levy, M.   Alpha heavy chain disease: A variant of Mediterranean lymphoma. *Arch. Intern. Med.* 128:432, 1971.

9 Lymphocytes

Ehrlich, one of the founders of modern hematology, denied the occurrence of lymphocytes in the bone marrow [4]. Studies of bone marrow sections obtained at autopsy, as well as from live patients, have proved this concept erroneous (Table 9-1).

Table 9-1. Incidence of Lymphoid Nodules in Bone Marrow: Review of Literature

Autopsy Studies			
1915	Askanazy [4]	34%	
1917	von Fischer [12]	62	
1939	Williams [44]	24	Age < 40 years
		39	Age > 40 years
1957	Hashimoto et al. [18]	34	
1960	Werner [43]	21	
1962	Lennert and Nagai [25]	36	
1967	Chomette et al. [7]	43	
In Vivo Studies			
1954	Johnstone (B) [21]	9	
1955	Pettet et al. (A) [34]	3	
1960	Rohr (A) [37]	4	
1964	Duhamel (B) [8]	1	
1968	Duhamel (B) [9]	3	
1974	Rywlin et al. (A) [39]	47	

(A) = aspiration; (B) = biopsy.

Source: From A. M. Rywlin, R. S. Ortega, and C. J. Dominguez, Lymphoid nodules of bone marrow: Normal and abnormal. *Blood* 43:389–400, 1974. By permission of Grune & Stratton.

It may be difficult for beginners to distinguish lymphocytes from normoblasts in hematoxylin and eosin-stained sections. Normoblasts have perfectly round, centrally located, darkly stained nuclei often surrounded by an artificial clear space. Lymphocytic nuclei are more irregular, exhibit more nuclear detail, and lack the circumferential perinuclear area (Fig. 9-1).

Normal Lymphoid Nodules

Lymphoid nodules have been the subject of very few clinical studies performed on aspirated or biopsied bone marrow. They have been found

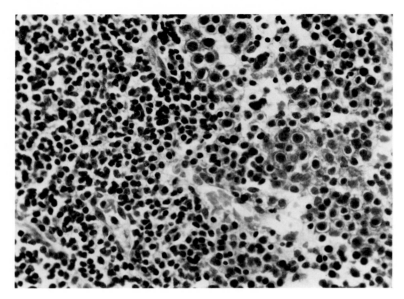

Figure 9-1
Comparative appearance of lymphocytes (*left half*) and nucleated red cells (*right half*). Note perinuclear clear area and almost perfectly round nuclei of red cells. (H&E, ×459.)

in from 1 to 47 percent of clinical specimens as compared to 21 to 62 percent of bone marrows obtained at autopsy (see Table 9-1). At the Mount Sinai Medical Center of Greater Miami, we have reviewed bone marrows from 400 consecutive cases in order to determine the incidence of lymphoid nodules in patients without a lymphoproliferative disorder [39]. Statistical data on these 400 patients are shown in Table 9-2.

Lymphoid nodules were present in 47 percent of bone marrow aspirates from patients without a lymphoproliferative disorder [39]. This incidence is much higher than the 9 percent reported by Johnstone [21], the highest published figure for in vivo studies. Our incidence is also high when compared to autopsy studies and is exceeded only by the 62 percent reported by von Fischer [12] (see Table 9-1). This high incidence of lymphoid nodules in our material is partly explained by the high average age of our hospital population (see Table 9-2). The discrepancy between our data and those reported in other in vivo studies is too high to be explained by age alone. The other in vivo studies show an incidence far below that found at autopsy, even in patients under 40 years of age (see Table 9-1). We are convinced that in addition to the high age of our population, the higher incidence in our material is due to our technic of aspirating more marrow and of concentrating the marrow particles by filtration (Chap. 1). It is of interest to note that the incidence of lymphoid nodules in our material, obtained by aspiration, is higher than that reported by biopsy technics (see Table 9-1).

Lymphoid nodules appear to be a normal or physiologic finding unrelated to any disease. They have been noted with approximately the same frequency in autopsies of healthy accident victims and of hospital patients [43]. The incidence of lymphoid nodules increases with advancing age, but they have been seen in patients of all ages. The average age of our patients with bone marrow lymphoid nodules was 71.9 years as compared with 63.5 years for patients without them (see Table 9-2). Sixty-one percent of our patients with lymphoid nodules were women, as contrasted with 48 percent women in the group without lymphoid nodules. This higher incidence of lymphoid nodules in women has been previously noted [7, 18] but has been denied by Werner [43].

Lymphoid nodules of bone marrow may be classified as follows.

Lymphoid Nodules (LN) of Bone Marrow

Normal
    Lymphoid follicles (LF)
    Lymphoid infiltrates (LI)
Abnormal
    Cytologically normal but increased number[a] or size[b] of lymphoid
        nodules—nodular lymphoid hyperplasia
        Predominantly LF
        Predominantly LI
        (Precursor of chronic lymphocytic leukemia or of malignant lym-
            phoma, small cell type)
    Cytologically abnormal
        Malignant lymphoma[c]
            Hodgkin's disease
            Intermediate cell type or lymphoblastic lymphoma
            Reticulum cell sarcoma (histiocytic lymphoma)
            Mixed cell lymphoma
    Granulomas

---

[a] Four or more LN per any lower power field (80 mm²).
[b] LN larger than 0.6 mm.
[c] May present with diffuse rather than nodular infiltrates.

Source: Modified from A. M. Rywlin, R. S. Ortega, and C. J. Dominguez, Lymphoid nodules of bone marrow: Normal and abnormal. *Blood* 43:389–400, 1974. By permission of Grune & Stratton.

With our technic of concentrating bone marrow particles by filtration, we accept up to 3 lymphoid nodules per low power field (eyepiece $10\times$, objective $4\times$, approximate area 80 mm²) as normal. Also, a normal lymphoid nodule should not exceed 0.6 mm in greatest dimension. Lymphoid nodules with abnormal cytologic features are abnormal regardless of density and size. The above criteria of normalcy are obviously arbitrary, and their significance is discussed below under Nodular Lymphoid Hyperplasia.

Table 9-2. Statistical Data

Patients without lymphoproliferative disorder	365	(100%)
With lymphoid nodules	173	(47%)
Females	105	(61%)
Males	68	(39%)
Average age: 71.9		
Without lymphoid nodules	192	(53%)
Females	92	(48%)
Males	100	(52%)
Average age: 63.5		
Patients with nodular lymphoid hyperplasia	10	
Females	8	
Males	2	
Average age: 74.5		
Patients with lymphoproliferative disorder	35	
Chronic lymphocytic leukemia	10	
Females	4	
Males	6	
Average age: 73.7		
Malignant lymphoma	25	
Females	15	
Males	10	
Average age: 62.6		
Hospital admissions (1972)	24,376	
Females	13,107	(54%)
Males	11,269	(46%)
Average age: 63.8		

Source: From A. M. Rywlin, R. S. Ortega, and C. J. Dominguez, Lymphoid nodules of bone marrow: Normal and abnormal. *Blood* 43:389–400, 1974. By permission of Grune & Stratton.

Table 9-3. Comparative Features of Lymphoid Follicles and Lymphoid Infiltrates

Feature	Lymphoid Follicles	Lymphoid Infiltrates
Shape	Round to oval	Irregular
Fat cells	Occasional at periphery	Usually preserved
Reticulum cells	Always present	Occasional and fewer
Blood vessels	Always present	Occasional
Reticulin framework	Organoid, distinctive	Normal to slightly accentuated
Germinal centers	5%	Never

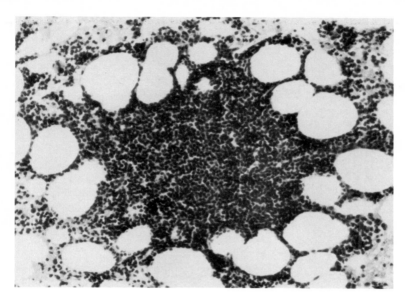

Figure 9-2
Sharply circumscribed lymphoid follicle with serrated edges formed by extension of lymphocytes between fat cells. (H&E, ×194.)

Normal lymphoid nodules measure from 0.08 to 0.6 mm in greatest dimension with an average of approximately 0.3 mm. They can be subdivided into two fairly distinct types: lymphoid follicles and lymphoid infiltrates (Table 9-3). About 84 percent of the lymphoid nodules are follicles and 16 percent are infiltrates. Lymphoid follicles resemble Malpighian follicles of the spleen. They are round to oval, often sharply circumscribed with serrated edges created by an extension of lymphocytes into spaces between fat cells (Fig. 9-2). Occasionally the circumscription may be less distinct (Fig. 9-3). Lymphoid follicles may display from 1 to 4 cross sections of small blood vessels, considered to represent precapillary arterioles. Sometimes the vessels are cut more longitudinally (Fig. 9-4). Lymphoid follicles are solid structures that contain no or only a few fat cells at the periphery and that are made up of sheets of small lymphocytes admixed with a few reticulum cells with a few plasma cells and mast cells toward the periphery (Fig. 9-5). Ten percent of the lymphoid follicles are surrounded by an increased number of eosinophils. Lipid granulomas are present in about 10 percent of the lymphoid follicles (Fig. 9-6; see Chap. 11). Five percent of lymphoid follicles exhibit well-developed germinal centers which may occasionally display hemorrhages and hyaline deposits (Figs. 9-7, 9-8). The reticulin framework of lymphoid follicles is accentuated when compared to the surrounding bone marrow and displays a characteristic pattern. The centers of the follicles contain a few radially oriented reticulin fibers,

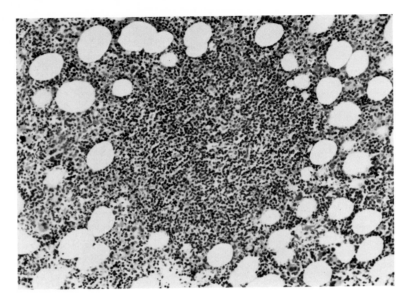

Figure 9-3
Less distinctly circumscribed lymphoid follicle. (H&E, ×154.)

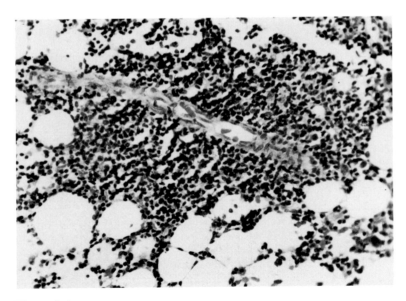

Figure 9-4
Lymphoid follicle oriented around longitudinally cut precapillary arteriole.
(H&E, ×264.)

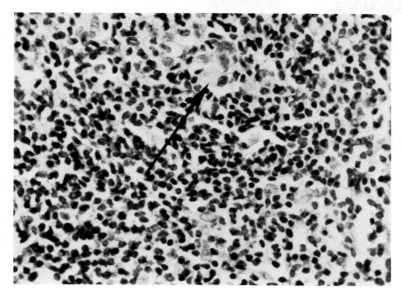

Figure 9-5
Cytology of lymphoid follicle. Paler, larger nuclei are reticulum cells (*arrow*).
Small dark nuclei are lymphocytes. (H&E, ×424.)

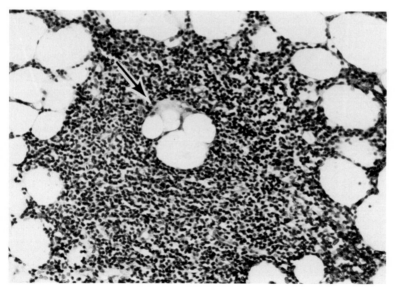

Figure 9-6
Lymphoid follicle with central lipid granuloma (*arrow*). (H&E, ×190.)

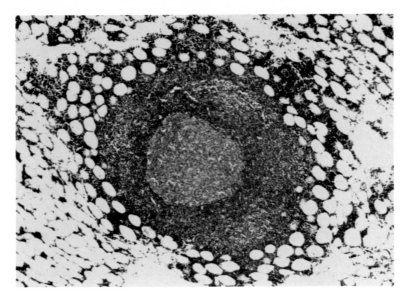

Figure 9-7
Lymphoid follicle with well-developed germinal center. (H&E, ×79.)

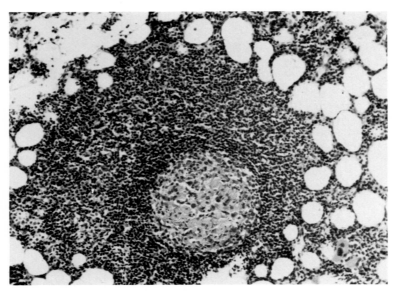

Figure 9-8
Hyaline deposit in germinal center of lymphoid follicle. (H&E, ×132.)

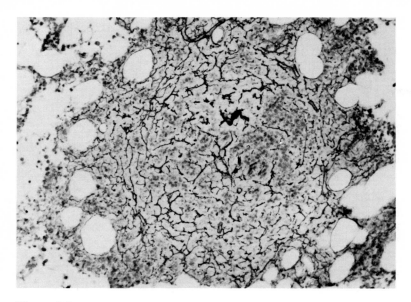

Figure 9-9
Reticulin framework of lymphoid follicle. Note centrofollicular vessels, tendency to radial position of central fibers, and concentric arrangement of peripheral fibers. (Gordon-Sweets', ×154.)

whereas the periphery shows a mesh or netlike arrangement of reticulin fibers created by the intersection of radial fibers with concentrically oriented peripheral fibers (Figs. 9-9, 9-10).

Lymphoid infiltrates are irregular in shape and usually display preserved fat cells (Fig. 9-11). When they are solid, the arrangement of the lymphocytes is looser and the circumscription is less sharp than in lymphoid follicles (Fig. 9-12). The reticulin framework of lymphoid infiltrates is normal or slightly accentuated when compared to normal hematopoietic or fatty marrow. A perivascular location of lymphoid infiltrates is noted occasionally. Cytologically, lymphoid infiltrates are composed of small lymphocytes with occasional reticulum cells, much fewer in number than in lymphoid follicles. Eosinophils and lipid granulomas are seen much less frequently in association with lymphoid infiltrates than with lymphoid follicles. Germinal centers are never seen in lymphoid infiltrates (see Table 9-3).

The number of lymphocytes in bone marrow smears does not accurately reflect the presence of lymphoid follicles. Occasionally, we have seen a smeared-out lymphoid nodule which mimicked chronic lymphocytic leukemia (CLL). Lymphoid infiltrates correlate somewhat better with smears than lymphoid follicles, possibly because of a lesser development of the reticulin framework in lymphoid infiltrates.

The subdivision of normal lymphoid nodules into follicles and infil-

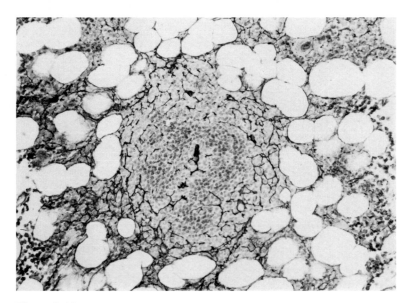

Figure 9-10
Reticulin framework of lymphoid follicle: formation of circumferential mesh and centrofollicular vessel. (Retic.-van Gieson, ×165.)

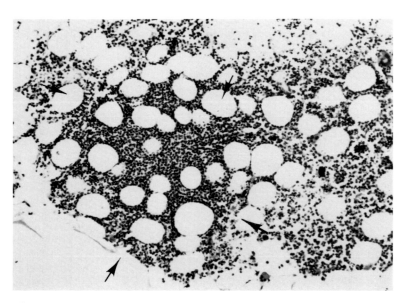

Figure 9-11
Lymphoid infiltrate (*between arrows*): poorly circumscribed, irregular in shape, and containing many fat cells. (H&E, ×132.)

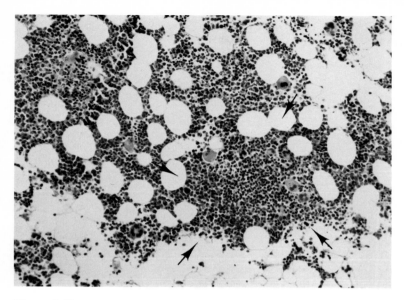

Figure 9-12
Lymphoid infiltrate (*between arrows*): a poorly circumscribed, loose aggregate of lymphocytes not containing any fat cells. (H&E, ×132.)

trates is essentially a simplification of the more elaborate classification of lymphoid nodules by Hashimoto et al. [18]. These authors distinguished four types of lymphoid nodules: (1) a nodule with a germinal center, (2) a sharply demarcated lymphoid nodule without a germinal center, (3) an ill-defined lymphoid nodule without a germinal center, and (4) a mere aggregate of lymphocytes. The first three types are lymphoid follicles with or without germinal centers, and the fourth is our lymphoid infiltrate. Transition stages seem to exist between lymphoid follicles and lymphoid infiltrates, and occasionally a sharp separation cannot be accomplished. It is entirely possible that some lymphoid infiltrates represent tangential sections of lymphoid follicles. The comparative features of lymphoid follicles and infiltrates are summarized in Table 9-3.

Nodular Lymphoid Hyperplasia (NLH)

We diagnose NLH when we can find a low power field (80 mm^2) containing 4 or more normal lymphoid nodules, or if any lymphoid nodule exceeds 0.6 mm in greatest dimension (Fig. 9-13). The density of lymphoid nodules is an imprecise criterion because it depends, to some extent, on how closely the bone marrow particles are packed during the embedding process. Cytologically and structurally the nodules in NLH have to be normal. The bone marrows of patients with

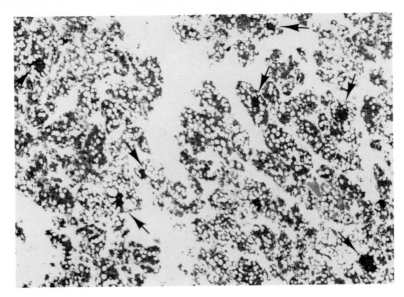

Figure 9-13
Nodular lymphoid hyperplasia of bone marrow in a 74-year-old woman with osteoarthritis and a Coombs-positive hemolytic anemia. The peripheral lymphocyte count was 2,800/mm³. The patient was lost to follow-up. In this very low power field, at least 8 lymphoid nodules can be counted (*arrows* point to 7 lymphoid nodules). (H&E, ×12.)

nodular lymphoid hyperplasia usually display both lymphoid follicles and lymphoid infiltrates; however, one or the other may predominate. The biologic and prognostic significance of nodular lymphoid hyperplasia is not understood at the present time. Prolonged clinical follow-up studies are necessary to evaluate this entity adequately. On the basis of our experience it appears that NLH of the follicular type may be present for many years without evolving into a malignant lymphoproliferative disorder. However, we have observed the transition of nodular lymphoid hyperplasia of the follicular type into a lymphoproliferative disorder on several occasions. Thus a 50-year-old woman with idiopathic cryoglobulinemia, thrombocytopenic purpura, splenomegaly, and a moderate monoclonal increase of IgM-kappa showed on bone marrow aspiration as many as 6 cytologically normal, normal-sized lymphoid follicles per low power field (Fig. 9-14A). Splenectomy performed at the same time revealed mild enlargement of Malpighian follicles. Two years later, biopsy of a hilar mass revealed malignant lymphoma of the intermediate cell type (see Non-Hodgkin's Lymphomas below). Nodules of malignant lymphoma, intermediate cell type, were found in a bone marrow aspirate performed at this time (Fig. 9-14B).

NLH of the follicular type can also be seen in association with rheu-

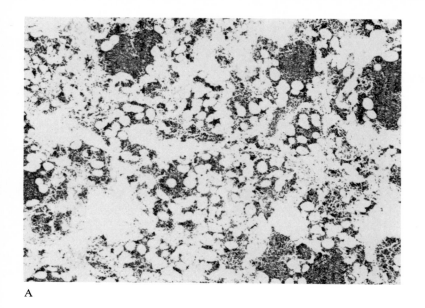

A

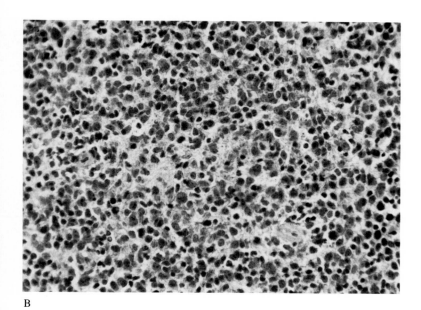

B

Figure 9-14
(A) Nodular lymphoid hyperplasia. Fifty-year-old woman with idiopathic cryoglobulinemia. Cytology of lymphoid nodules is quite normal. (H&E, ×49.) (B) Same patient as in A. Bone marrow two years later shows nodules of intermediate cell (prolymphocytic, poorly differentiated lymphocytic) lymphoma. (H&E, ×308.)

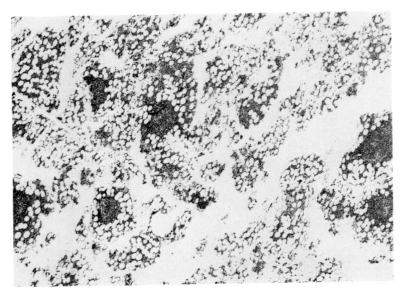

Figure 9-15
Nodular lymphoid hyperplasia of bone marrow in a patient with established Hodgkin's disease. (H&E, ×21.)

matoid arthritis, hyperthyroidism, hemolytic anemia, and malignant lymphomas. We have seen it in patients with documented reticulum cell sarcoma and Hodgkin's disease (Fig. 9-15). Obviously, the NLH in these cases does not represent involvement of the bone marrow by lymphoma because the cytology of the nodules is quite different from the lymphomas. NLH in Hodgkin's disease is best interpreted as a nonspecific reaction of the marrow, similar to granulocytic, megakaryocytic, or eosinophilic hyperplasia. It is unlikely that NLH of the bone marrow in cases of Hodgkin's disease represents a precursor state of a small cell lymphoma or chronic lymphocytic leukemia because we have observed it too often and it has been reported by others [13, 28]. However, this latter interpretation of NLH in cases of Hodgkin's disease remains a possibility.

If NLH of the bone marrow is encountered in a patient with a malignant small cell lymphoma diagnosed elsewhere in the body, it must be interpreted with the utmost caution. At the present stage of our knowledge, it may be difficult to decide whether one is dealing with actual marrow involvement by a small cell lymphoma or with NLH. Confluence, irregular shape, tendency to fragmentation, increased size of the lymphoid nodules, and above all, the presence of increased numbers of intermediate lymphocytes and lymphoblasts would be convincing arguments in favor of a malignant lymphoma. Giemsa-stained sections are essential for the recognition of lymphoblasts. The position of lymphoid

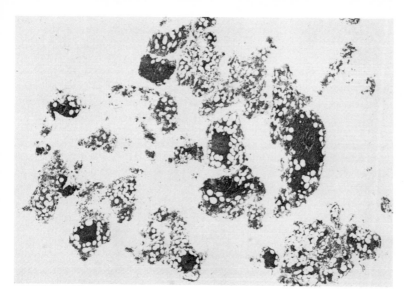

Figure 9-16
Sixty-eight-year-old woman with mild anemia and normal peripheral blood lymphocytes. Three years later, bone marrow and peripheral blood were unchanged. Diagnostic considerations: NLH, small cell lymphoma of bone marrow, or precursor stage of CLL. (H&E, ×21.)

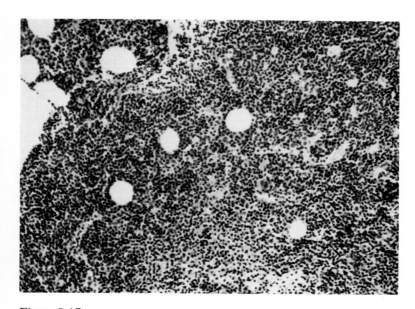

Figure 9-17
Chronic lymphocytic leukemia. Diffuse infiltration of marrow with lymphocytes with extensive replacement of fat cells. Seventy-three-year-old man with peripheral blood lymphocytosis of 45,000/mm³. (H&E, ×154.)

109

nodules with respect to bone trabeculae does not always help in the separation of normal from lymphomatous lymphoid nodules because both can occur in close proximity to bone [12] and can extend along endosteal surfaces of trabeculae. However, massive peritrabecular lymphocytic infiltration is seen only in malignant lymphomas. Eosinophils and plasma cells may be associated with normal as well as with lymphomatous lymphoid nodules. The reticulin pattern of normal and lymphomatous lymphoid nodules may be identical (compare Figs. 9-10 and 9-24).

NLH of the infiltrate type is equally difficult to interpret. The difference between NLH of the infiltrate type and fully developed CLL is quantitative rather than qualitative. When the nodular infiltrates become confluent, the diagnosis of a small cell lymphocytic proliferative disorder is obvious. NLH of the infiltrate type probably represents a precursor state of CLL or of a small cell lymphoma. We do not have enough cases with adequate follow-up to corroborate this hypothesis. At the present time, when faced with a case of NLH of the follicular or the infiltrate type, we recommend periodic follow-up studies.

The incubation period of CLL or small cell malignant lymphoma may be very long. Rappaport [35] reported a patient with an excessive number of bone marrow lymphoid nodules who was followed for seven years before a sustained moderate peripheral blood lymphocytosis became evident. Similarly, Figure 9-16 depicts the bone marrow of a 68-year-old woman with mild anemia and a normal white blood cell count. She had no lymphadenopathy or hepatosplenomegaly. A repeat bone marrow aspiration three years later showed an identical pattern, still without peripheral blood lymphocytosis. Unfortunately, this patient was lost to follow-up. The diagnostic considerations on this marrow were NLH, small cell lymphoma of bone marrow, or pre-CLL.

NLH, though defined by arbitrary and imprecise criteria, has to be recognized as an entity when attempts are being made to stage malignant lymphomas. Only meticulous follow-up studies with good clinicopathologic correlations will produce a sharp distinction between NLH and small cell lymphoproliferative disorders.

Chronic Lymphocytic Leukemia (CLL)

Four distinct patterns of bone marrow infiltrates can be seen in patients with CLL: diffuse, nodular, interstitial, and mixed diffuse and nodular (Figs. 9-17, 9-18, 9-19). The mixed type is seen most frequently; the pure nodular and interstitial types are rarest. In the interstitial type of infiltrate the fat cells are well preserved. The lymphoid infiltrates are in the tissue spaces separating fat cells. They replace the hematopoietic elements which are normally located between the fat cells. In the other types of lymphocytic infiltration in CLL, there is replacement of hematopoietic as well as fatty marrow by lymphocytes, resulting in solid collections of lymphocytes without any fat cells. This replacement of

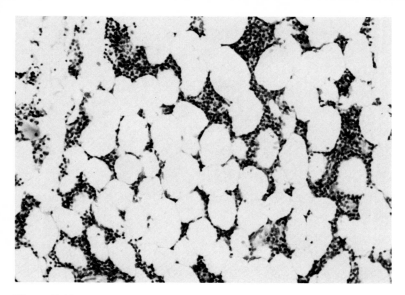

Figure 9-18
Chronic lymphocytic leukemia. Interstitial lymphoid infiltrates with good preservation of fat cells. Eighty-year-old man with peripheral blood lymphocytosis of 14,000/mm³. (H&E, ×154.)

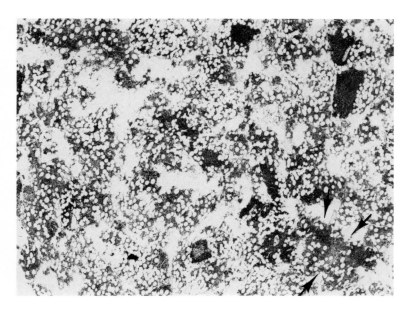

Figure 9-19
Chronic lymphocytic leukemia. Predominantly nodular and some diffuse infiltration (*arrows*) of marrow with lymphocytes. Eighty-two-year-old woman with peripheral blood lymphocytosis of 3,450/mm³. (H&E, ×19.)

111

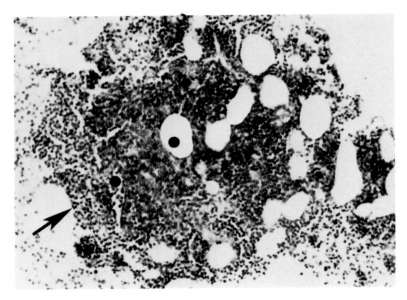

Figure 9-20
Chronic lymphocytic leukemia. Small lymphocytes (*arrow*) surrounding intermediate lymphocytes and lymphoblasts (*between dots*). (Giemsa, ×182.)

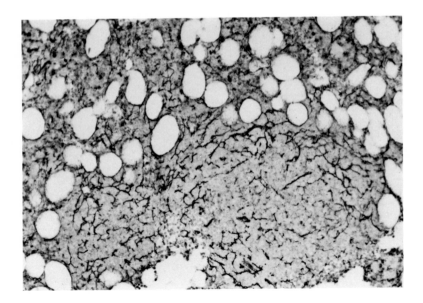

Figure 9-21
Chronic lymphocytic leukemia. Same patient as in Figure 9-19. Increased reticulin framework in nodules (*lower right half*) as well as in areas of diffuse infiltration (*upper left corner*). (Gordon-Sweets', ×154.)

fatty and hematopoietic elements may occur in a diffuse, nodular, or mixed pattern. Cytologically, the infiltrates are made up of small lymphocytes; however, in contrast to NLH, an increased number of intermediate lymphocytes and lymphoblasts is invariably present (Fig. 9-20).

The reticulin framework of the marrow is accentuated in the involved areas in the majority of cases (Fig. 9-21). The origin of these fibers is not entirely clear. The number of reticulum cells present in the lymphoid infiltrate cannot possibly account for the number of reticulin fibers. At least some of the reticulin fibers seem to be derived from replaced fat cells which are normally surrounded by circular reticulin fibers [25, 26].

Malignant Lymphomas

By convention and somewhat arbitrarily, the term *malignant lymphoma* is used collectively for only some of the neoplastic proliferations of lymphocytes, monocytes (reticulum cells, histiocytes), and plasma cells listed below.

Neoplastic Proliferations of Lymphocytes, Monocytes (Reticulum Cells, Histiocytes), and Plasma Cells

---

Hodgkin's disease
Lymphocytic lymphomas, follicular and diffuse
Lymphocytic leukemias
Histiocytic lymphoma (reticulum cell sarcoma)
Reticuloses
Monocytic leukemias
Burkitt's tumor
Mycosis fungoides
Multiple myeloma
Waldenström's macroglobulinemia
Heavy-chain disease: alpha, Mediterranean lymphoma (Seligman's disease); gamma, Franklin's disease; mu-chain disease

---

Malignant lymphoma includes Hodgkin's disease, lymphocytic lymphomas, reticulum cell sarcoma (histiocytic lymphoma), Burkitt's tumor, and mycosis fungoides. These neoplasms tend to be localized and present as a dominant mass at the time of diagnosis. Malignant lymphomas arise primarily, but not exclusively, in lymph nodes. However, Burkitt's tumor usually occurs outside of lymph nodes, and mycosis fungoides is primarily a cutaneous neoplasm.

Hematopoietic and lymphoreticular malignancies exhibit a unique feature among malignant neoplasms: a tendency to multicentricity and systemic involvement with or without a leukemic blood picture. Systemic involvement has to be distinguished from widespread metastases. Metastases usually form grossly visible nodules which may involve many different tissues, whereas systemic involvement tends to be diffuse and limited to organs normally housing hematopoietic and lymphoreticular tissues. Transition stages among a localized tumor mass, systemic involvement, and leukemia exist for neoplasias of lymphocytes, reticulum cells, plasma cells, granulocytes, and mast cells. Transition stages between lymphoma and leukemia are sometimes called *leukosarcoma*. Tumors formed by immature granulocytes are known as *chloromas* or *granulocytic sarcomas* [35]. Proliferative disorders of histiocytes are listed below. Localized, multicentric, or systemic, they are reactive (inflammatory) or neoplastic. The bone marrow is often involved in the proliferative disorders of histiocytes.

Proliferative Disorders of Histiocytes
(Reticulum cells, Macrophages, Monocytes)

Localized
    Reactive or inflammatory: granulomatous inflammation
    Neoplastic
        Benign: e.g., fibrous histiocytoma, giant cell reticulohistiocytoma
        Malignant: e.g., malignant fibrous histiocytoma
    Uncertain whether reactive or neoplastic: e.g., juvenile xanthogranuloma, xanthoma
Multicentric or generalized
    Reactive or inflammatory: e.g., generalized military tuberculosis, sarcoidosis
    Neoplastic
        Eosinophilic granuloma, Hand-Schüller-Christian disease, histiocytic lymphoma (reticulum cell sarcoma)
Systemic (reticulosis, histiocytosis, reticuloendotheliosis)
    Reactive
        Storage diseases: Gaucher's disease, Niemann-Pick disease, ceroid histiocytosis
    Neoplastic
        Letterer-Siwe disease
        Histiocytic medullary reticulosis
        Leukemic reticulosis
            Monocytic leukemia
            Leukemic reticuloendotheliosis (hairy cell leukemia)

Non-Hodgkin's Lymphomas
To date there is no generally accepted classification for non-Hodgkin's lymphomas. Virchow coined the term *lymphosarcoma* for primary malignant neoplasms arising in lymph nodes. Virchow's lymphosarcomas were composed of small or large cells. Later pathologists expressed the view that large cell lymphosarcomas were derived from endothelial cells, retothelial cells, or reticulum cells [11, 33, 37]. Terms such as *endothelial sarcoma, retothelial sarcoma,* and *reticulum cell*

sarcoma were introduced to describe the large cell lymphosarcoma. Of these terms *reticulum cell sarcoma* became the most popular. Another type of malignant lymphoma was described by Baehr and Klemperer [5] as *giant follicle lymphoblastoma*. The difficulty of distinguishing this entity from reactive follicular hyperplasia, its relatively good prognosis as compared to other lymphomas, and its tendencies to develop a diffuse growth pattern and to lose its nodular appearance were all recognized.

The above outlined classification of malignant lymphomas (lymphosarcoma, reticulum cell sarcoma, giant follicular lymphoblastoma) coexisted with another classification based on the application of conventional cytologic, hematologic nomenclature to Giemsa-stained histologic sections. According to this view, the small mature lymphocyte is the result of maturation of the lymphoblast, a large cell with a round to oval nucleus, prominent nucleoli, a large nuclear to cytoplasmic ratio, and a dark blue rim of cytoplasm with the Giemsa stain. The intermediate stage between the mature small lymphocyte and the lymphoblast is the prolymphocyte. Malignant lymphomas were therefore divided into the small lymphocytic, the prolymphocytic, and the lymphoblastic types. The large cell lymphomas that failed to reveal the characteristic cytologic features of lymphoblasts were called reticulum cell sarcomas.

These classifications were gradually replaced by Rappaport's classification (see list) [35]. The Rappaport classification is simple and fairly well reproducible, and it has proved prognostically significant. There is, however, increasing evidence that it is histogenetically incorrect.

Rappaport's Classification of Malignant Lymphomas (ML) [35]
(All of these may occur in a nodular or a diffuse form.)

Lymphocytic type, well differentiated
Lymphocytic type, poorly differentiated
Histiocytic—lymphocytic type
Histiocytic type
Undifferentiated type

The Rappaport classification is based on the assumption that germinal center cell lymphomas do not exist and that all lymphomas may exhibit a nodular or a diffuse growth pattern [36]. Recent investigators have contradicted this view and have presented evidence that nodular (follicular) lymphomas arise from or develop into germinal center lymphocytes [20, 24, 27, 30]. Also, the substitution of histiocytic lymphoma for reticulum cell sarcoma does not appear justified. The term *histiocyte* was introduced by Aschoff and Kiyono [2, 3] to denote that the wandering macrophage was of tissue origin rather than of peripheral blood origin as believed by Metchnikoff. Modern investigators consider the wandering macrophage to be derived from monocytes arriving from the bone marrow via the peripheral blood [16]. Furthermore, it is not really possible to decide by histologic examination whether a neoplasm is derived from reticulum cells (fixed macrophages) or histiocytes (wandering macrophages). Also, many of the large cell malignant lymphomas appear to be derived from lymphoid cells rather than from reticulum cells or histiocytes.

Modern studies have divided lymphocytes into B and T populations [17]. The responses of B and T lymphocytes to antigens and mitogens have been studied and applied to events observed in lymph nodes. The stimulated small lymphocytes enlarge and give rise to immunoblasts. Rappaport's terminology of referring to larger lymphoid cells as poorly differentiated appears inappropriate because from a functional point of view these cells are more differentiated. The stimulated B lymphocyte seems to move into the germinal center, where it enlarges and its nucleus becomes cleaved. Eventually the stimulated lymphocyte acquires prominent nucleoli and a dark blue rim of cytoplasm demonstrable with the Giemsa stain. This cytoplasm, being rich in RNA, is also pyroninophilic, and is called *germinoblast* by Lennert [23, 24]. The germinoblast appears to have two options: (1) it can become a lymphoblast and can participate in lymphopoiesis, or (2) it can become an immunoblast and evolve into an immunoglobulin-producing plasma cell (see Fig. 9-22).

In spite of the diversity of terms proposed for the non-Hodgkin's lymphomas, there is general agreement that these lymphomas may exhibit a follicular or a diffuse growth pattern and that they may be composed of small, intermediate, or large cells. Based on these two observations we use the classification on page 117. Most of the large cell lymphomas exhibit round nuclei with prominent nucleoli and a rim of well-defined cytoplasm which is basophilic with the Giemsa stain and pyroninophilic with the methyl green–pyronine reaction. These tumors we call *blastic lymphomas* (Plate IIIB). We do not believe that it is possible, at the present time, to distinguish accurately germinoblasts, immunoblasts, and lymphoblasts in neoplastic processes. Other large cell lymphomas with more pleomorphic and bizarre nuclei, without a basophilic and pyroninophilic rim of cytoplasm, we call *reticulum cell sarcomas* (*histiocytic lymphoma*) (Plate IIIA). It should be noted that with hematoxylin and eosin-stained sections, it may be impossible to differentiate reticulum cells (histiocytes) from blasts.

Because we cannot distinguish the enlarged stimulated lymphocyte on its way to becoming an immunoblast from the prolymphocyte, i.e., the maturing lymphoblasts evolving into a small lymphocyte (Fig. 9-22), we have chosen the noncommittal term *intermediate lymphocyte* to denote this cell type. This term is identical with the cleaved cell of Lukes and Collins [30] and the germinocyte of Lennert [24].

The exact frequency of bone marrow involvement in malignant lymphomas is unknown. We have demonstrated bone marrow involvement in 11 out of 25 consecutive patients with malignant lymphomas [39]. This incidence is rather high and is partly a result of performing bone marrow aspirations in lymphoma patients clinically suspected of having bone marrow involvement, rather than performing them routinely in all patients with lymphoma. Also, with our technic more marrow is obtained

Follicular lymphomas (1)
    Intermediate cell type (2)

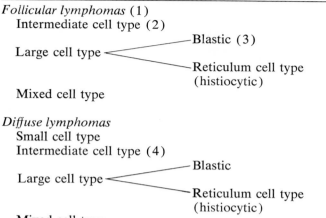

    Large cell type ——— Blastic (3)
                    ——— Reticulum cell type
                         (histiocytic)
    Mixed cell type

Diffuse lymphomas
    Small cell type
    Intermediate cell type (4)

    Large cell type ——— Blastic
                    ——— Reticulum cell type
                         (histiocytic)
    Mixed cell type

1. Follicular lymphomas exhibit a nodular growth pattern and originate from or differentiate into germinal center cells.
2. This is the cleaved cell of Lukes and Collins [30] or the germinocyte of Lennert [24]; (see Fig. 9-22); a follicular lymphoma made
   up of small, round, "mature" lymphocytes has not been described.
3. Identification of "blasts" is based on the presence of narrow, blue
   rims of cytoplasm with the Giemsa stain in association with
   prominent nucleoli; the cytoplasm is also pyroninophilic.
4. This is the germinal center cell described under (2); however, the
   growth pattern is diffuse.

than with needle biopsy or clot section methods. It is quite possible that
the aspiration of bone marrow by our technic at two or three sites might
reveal a higher incidence of marrow involvement by lymphoma than
open surgical biopsy of marrow performed at one site.

Bone marrow involvement by lymphoma may be nodular or diffuse.
Nodular involvement is more frequent (Figs. 9-23, 9-24). No conclusions can be drawn from this observation as to the growth pattern of the
lymphoma in lymph nodes. Diffuse lymphomas involve the marrow
more frequently in a nodular fashion. The nodules occasionally are very
regular, round, and almost equal in size (see Fig. 9-23A). It seems to
be a property of lymphoid cells to grow in such uniform, round nodules,
because such nodules are never formed by carcinomas or by reticulum
cell sarcomas. In the non-Hodgkin's lymphomas, the lymphomatous bone
marrow nodules are cytologically identical with the original lymphoma.
In blastic lymphoma and in reticulum cell sarcoma the lymphomatous
bone marrow nodules are easily distinguishable from normal lymphoid
nodules. The cytology of the nodules is quite different from normal
lymphoid nodules (Fig. 9-23B). A lymphoblast cannot be easily distinguished from a myeloblast, and therefore it is difficult to separate a

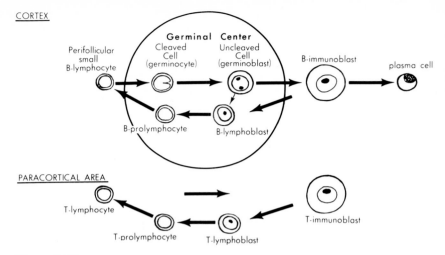

Figure 9-22
Postulated relationships between lymphoid cells in cortical and paracortical regions of lymph nodes. In my opinion, germinoblasts, immunoblasts, and lymphoblasts cannot be reliably distinguished at the present time, particularly in neoplastic processes.

blastic lymphoma/leukemia from a myeloblastic sarcoma/leukemia (chloroma, granulocytic sarcoma). The distinction can be accomplished by looking for more mature cells accompanying the blasts. For the identification of myeloblasts the finding of eosinophilic and neutrophilic myelocytes is particularly useful. Neutrophilic granules can be easily demonstrated in formalin-fixed, paraffin-embedded tissue sections by the AS-D-chloracetate esterase reaction of Leder [22] (see Appendix, 5). If one deals with lymphoblastic nodules, the myelocytes are pushed aside and are seen primarily in the marrow surrounding the lymphomatous nodules (Plate IC, D). In early myeloblastic leukemia the marrow involvement is spotty. The collections of myeloblasts are never as discrete and as round as the lymphoblastic collections. The neutrophilic myelocytes are seen throughout the myeloblastic foci.

Lymphoid nodules in the bone marrow of patients with an established diagnosis of malignant lymphoma of the small lymphocytic type must be interpreted with utmost care. They are discussed under Nodular Lymphoid Hyperplasia.

It is occasionally difficult to decide whether a collection of foreign cells in the bone marrow represents reticulum cell sarcoma or undifferentiated carcinoma. The production of mucin by the cells as evidenced by a positive mucicarmine stain and a grouping of cells as shown by a reticulin stain are arguments in favor of carcinoma.

A mixed follicular malignant lymphoma involving the bone marrow is

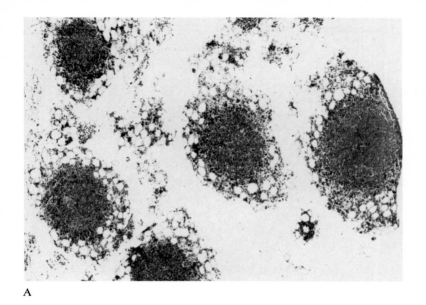

A

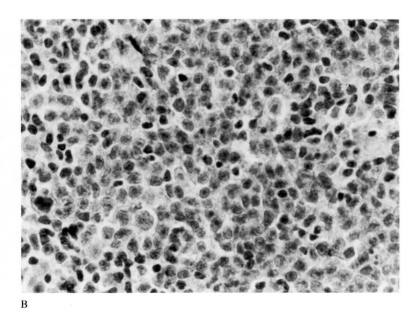

B

Figure 9-23
(A) Nodules of blastic lymphoma. Note uniform, round shape of nodules.
(H&E, ×49.) (B) Same case as in A. Blasts resemble reticulum cells in
H&E-stained sections. (H&E, ×494.)

119

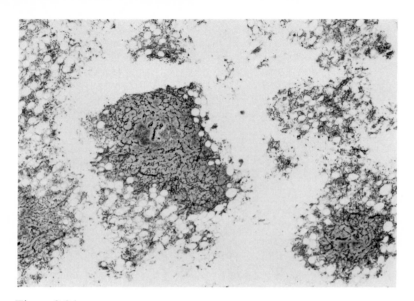

Figure 9-24
Same case as in Figure 9-23. Reticulin framework of lymphomatous nodules is very similar to framework of normal lymphoid nodules. (Gordon-Sweets', ×49.)

illustrated by the following case: A 65-year-old man with hepatospleno-megaly, mild anemia, and a monoclonal IgM-lambda gammopathy showed numerous lymphoid nodules imitating germinal centers in a bone marrow aspirate (Fig. 9-25A). Because of the similarity to germi-nal centers, a diagnosis of lymphoma was not made until a liver biopsy revealed similar lymphoid nodules in the portal spaces (Fig. 9-25B). These lymphomatous nodules resembled germinal centers and were made up of small, intermediate, and blastic lymphocytes. Another ex-ample of a mixed follicular lymphoma, not imitating a germinal center, is pictured in Figure 9-26.

Hodgkin's Disease

In contrast to the non-Hodgkin's lymphomas, there is almost universal acceptance of the Rye classification of Hodgkin's disease into (1) lymphocyte-predominance type; (2) nodular sclerosis type; (3) mixed cellularity type; and (4) lymphocyte-depletion type [31].

In Hodgkin's disease the marrow may show a nonspecific reaction pattern including nodular lymphoid, granulocytic, eosinophilic, mega-karyocytic, or plasma cellular hyperplasia. Occasionally, sarcoidlike granulomas are found. These should not be interpreted as involvement of the marrow by Hodgkin's disease. Actual involvement of the marrow

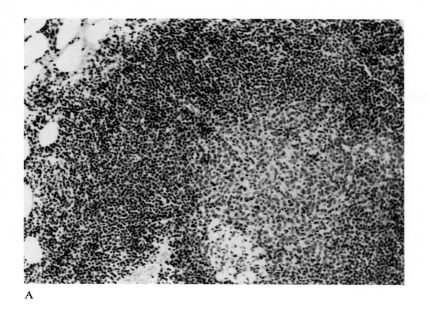

A

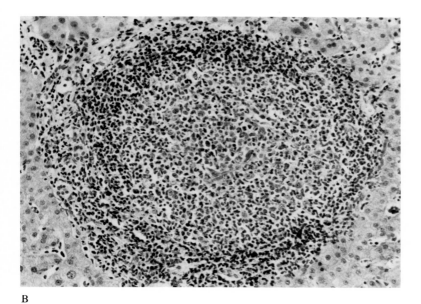

B

Figure 9-25
(A) Mixed follicular lymphoma imitating germinal center in a patient with monoclonal macroglobulinemia. The lymphoma is made up of small, intermediate, and large lymphocytes. (H&E, ×132.) (B) Same patient as in A. Mixed follicular lymphoma of liver. (H&E, ×166.)

121

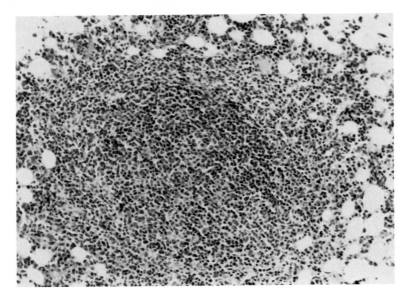

Figure 9-26
Mixed follicular lymphoma not imitating germinal center. (H&E, ×132.)

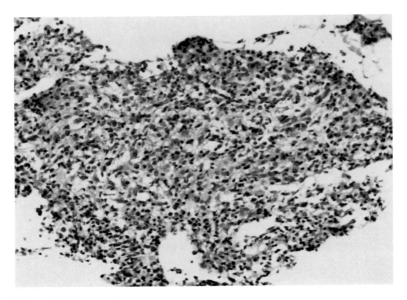

Figure 9-27
Atypical lymphoreticular nodule of marrow in a patient with Hodgkin's disease. This nodule is quite different from a normal lymphoid nodule and is consistent with Hodgkin's disease. Note fibrosis. (H&E, ×45.)

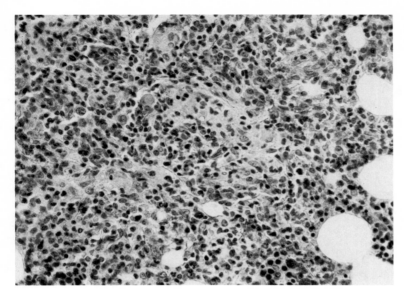

Figure 9-28
Atypical lymphoreticular nodule of marrow consistent with Hodgkin's disease. Note tendency to elongation of histiocytes and presence of fibroblasts. (H&E, ×308.)

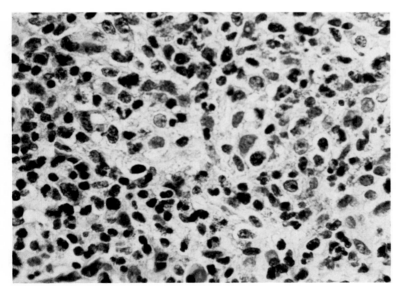

Figure 9-29
Atypical lymphoreticular nodule of marrow consistent with Hodgkin's disease. Note atypical appearance of histiocytes. (H&E, ×459.)

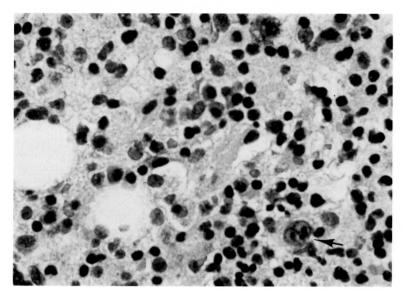

Figure 9-30
Lymphoreticular nodule of marrow diagnostic of Hodgkin's disease. Note
Reed-Sternberg cell (*arrow*). (H&E, ×492.)

by Hodgkin's disease may be of two types: (1) diagnostic of Hodgkin's disease, when typical Reed-Sternberg cells are present; and (2) consistent with Hodgkin's disease, when atypical lymphoreticular nodules without characteristic Reed-Sternberg cells are found. When such nodules are present in the bone marrow in a patient with proved Hodgkin's disease elsewhere, the marrow should be considered involved by Hodgkin's disease. If such nodules are seen in a patient in whom a diagnosis of Hodgkin's disease has not been established, they should be interpreted as suggestive of Hodgkin's disease.

The involvement of the bone marrow in Hodgkin's disease is more often nodular than diffuse. The nodules are made up of atypical reticulum cells admixed with lymphocytes, eosinophils, plasma cells, and invariably a few fibroblasts (Figs. 9-27 to 9-29). The reticulin framework of these nodules is increased. When Reed-Sternberg cells are present, the nodules are diagnostic of Hodgkin's disease (Fig. 9-30). When Reed-Sternberg cells cannot be demonstrated, the differential diagnoses include mixed lymphoma and certain granulomas. The presence of fibrosis and eosinophils speaks in favor of Hodgkin's disease rather than of mixed lymphoma.

The eosinophilic fibrohistiocytic lesion and drug-related granulomas (Chap. 11) are distinguished from Hodgkin's disease by the absence of atypism in the histiocytes.

Lymphocyte-depletion Hodgkin's disease of the Rye classification [31] encompasses the diffuse fibrosis and reticular types of the Lukes-Butler-Hicks classification [29]. Diffuse fibrosis, more correctly called *diffuse hyalinosis,* shows few diagnostic Reed-Sternberg cells. When diffuse or nodular hyaline deposits are found in the bone marrow, amyloidosis, paramyloidosis, sarcoidosis, and diffuse "fibrosis" type of Hodgkin's disease have to be considered. Amyloidosis can be confirmed by the proper stains. In paramyloidosis only some of the stains for amyloid are positive, and there may be a foreign-body giant cell reaction around the hyaline deposits. In sarcoidosis the hyaline deposits are nodular, and more characteristic sarcoid granulomas can be found. In Hodgkin's disease the hyaline deposits are confluent, and some atypical reticulum cells and an occasional Reed-Sternberg cell are seen. Lymphocyte-depletion Hodgkin's disease of the reticular type may show hyalinosis in association with many bizarre reticulum cells and pleomorphic Reed-Sternberg cells.

Lymphocyte-depletion Hodgkin's disease presents clinically as an acute febrile illness associated with pancytopenia, lymphocytopenia, signs of hepatic dysfunction, and frequent absence of peripheral lymphadenopathy. There is a tendency to an infradiaphragmatic distribution of the lesions and to extensive bone marrow involvement [32].

Leukemic Reticuloendotheliosis (LRE)

Leukemic reticuloendotheliosis has been described in the literature under a variety of terms: hairy cell leukemia [15]; lymphoid myelofibrosis [10]; chronic myelosclerosis, lymphoid type [42]; medullary and splenic histiolymphocytosis [14]; and histiolymphocytic reticulosis with myelofibrosis [1]. *Lymphoid myelofibrosis* is the best descriptive term for the pathologic findings in the bone marrow. Clinically the disease is characterized by an insidious onset, with marked splenomegaly, inconspicuous peripheral lymphadenopathy, and pancytopenia with lymphocytosis. In the peripheral blood, mononuclear cells with irregular, hairlike cytoplasmic projections are particularly clearly seen with phase microscopy. These cells contain a tartrate-resistant acid phosphatase isoenzyme [45]. They also exhibit ultrastructurally characteristic cytoplasmic inclusions, the ribosome-lamellar complexes [15], which can be recognized with the light microscope in Giemsa-stained smears as rod-shaped inclusions. These inclusions are pyroninophilic.

Bone marrow aspirations in LRE usually result in a dry tap. Bone marrow biopsies show a diffuse increase in reticulin fibers associated with a diffuse but loose infiltration with cells resembling lymphocytes (Fig. 9-31). Osteosclerosis has not been reported.

There is no general agreement, at the present time, whether the proliferating cells belong to the lymphoid or monocytic series [6, 19].

Serum protein electrophoretic patterns are either normal or show hyperglobulinemia. Macroglobulinemia has not been reported.

Macroglobulinemia

The bone marrow does not present a uniform histologic picture in cases of monoclonal macroglobulinemia [40]. A high index of suspicion and serum and urine protein electrophoresis and immunoelectrophoresis in all patients with a lymphoreticular proliferative disorder are the best ways to diagnose macroglobulinemia. We have observed a spectrum of histologic findings in the bone marrow of patients with monoclonal macroglobulinemia [40] including normal lymphoid nodules, nodular lymphoid hyperplasia, follicular malignant lymphomas, diffuse infiltration of the marrow with lymphocytes with or without a leukemic blood picture, and the absence of lymphoid collections. The malignant lymphomas involving the bone marrow and associated with macroglobulinemia included blastic and intermediate cell types and mixed follicular lymphoma (see Fig. 9-25A). Macroglobulinemia can also be associated with generalized amyloidosis. In one such case the bone marrow showed normal lymphoid nodules. No evidence of a malignant lymphoma could be found at autopsy.

Rarely monoclonal macroglobulinemia may be associated with a morphologic picture which is identical with multiple myeloma. Bone marrow fibrosis has also been reported in macroglobulinemia [37]. Monoclonal macroglobulinemia is seen in patients with cold agglutinin disease, in which the marrow may show a slight increase in plasma cells. We have also observed monoclonal macroglobulinemia in a patient with cryoglobulinemia. The bone marrow in this patient at first showed nodular lymphoid hyperplasia and later nodular infiltration with intermediate cell type lymphoma (see Fig. 9-14).

Other morphologic features of the bone marrow in macroglobulinemia include plasmacytoid lymphocytes and increased numbers of mast cells, Dutcher bodies, PAS-positive material in blood vessel walls and in lymphoid nodules, as well as PAS-positive intravascular plasma and extravascular lake-like and linear precipitates (Table 9-4; Figs. 9-32, 9-33, 9-34; Plate IIC, D). Plasmacytoid lymphocytes represent morphologically an intermediate stage between lymphocytes and plasma cells. Dutcher bodies are PAS-positive intranuclear inclusions (Plate IIA). Plasmacytoid lymphocytes and Dutcher bodies can be seen outside of macroglobulinemia. We have described a new inclusion which consists of an eosinophilic, PAS-positive material, apparently intranuclear, divided by thin, spidery strands of chromatin (Plate IIB) [40]. We have observed this peculiar inclusion in cases of monoclonal and polyclonal macroglobulinemia as well as in malignant lymphomas associated with an IgA monoclonal gammopathy. It may represent a variant of a Dutcher body.

In a study of 26 cases of monoclonal macroglobulinemia, we concluded that even though the average macroglobulin levels were higher in patients with abnormal lymphoid infiltrates in the bone marrow than in those with normal or no lymphoid collections, there was considerable

Table 9-4. Monoclonal Macroglobulinemia: Histologic Features of Bone Marrow (26 patients)

Histologic Features	No. Patients
1. Increased plasma cells[a]	26
2. Plasmacytoid lymphocytes	26
3. Increased mast cells[a]	11
4. PAS + extravascular material	14
5. PAS + intravascular plasma	14
6. PAS + blood vessel walls	14
7. Dutcher bodies	10
8. Variants of Dutcher bodies	14
9. Hypercellular marrow[b]	10
10. Hypocellular marrow	2
11. Increased megakaryocytes	4
12. Erythroblastic hyperplasia	10
13. Megaloblastosis	1
14. Ringed sideroblasts	1
15. Increased hemosiderin	3
16. Decreased hemosiderin	18
17. Granulocytic hyperplasia	2
18. Eosinophilia	7
19. Increased reticulin fibers	10

[a] In some cases the increase was focal in association with lymphoid collections.
[b] Hypercellularity was evaluated outside of lymphoid infiltrates.

Source: Reprinted with permission from A. M. Rywlin, F. Civantos, R. S. Ortega, and C. J. Dominguez, Bone marrow histology in monoclonal macroglobulinemia. *American Journal of Clinical Pathology* 63:769, 1975.

overlap among individual patients in the different groups [40]. Similarly, no correlation between macroglobulin levels and other histologic features could be established. Patients with monoclonal macroglobulinemia include benign monoclonal gammopathy, various lymphoproliferative disorders of the bone marrow, nodal or extranodal lymphomas, and carcinomas. It is doubtful whether Waldenström's macroglobulinemia should be separated from this spectrum by the two criteria which have been proposed: an arbitrary minimum macroglobulin level and the presence of a "lymphoid infiltrate" of the bone marrow [41]. The considerable overlap of macroglobulin levels among patients with the different types of lymphoid infiltrates prohibits the choice of a rational minimum level. Also, the term *lymphoid infiltrate* is too vague, because different types of lymphoid infiltrates, or even no lymphoid infiltrates, may be seen in the marrow of patients with monoclonal macroglobulinemia.

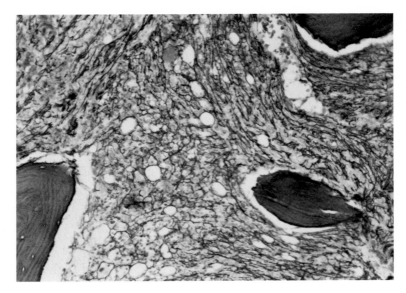

Figure 9-31
Leukemic reticuloendotheliosis. Sixty-seven-year-old woman with spleno-megaly, pancytopenia, and "dry taps" on bone marrow aspiration. Dense mesh of reticulin fibers. Majority of the cells infiltrating the bone marrow are lymphoid in appearance. (H&E, ×174.)

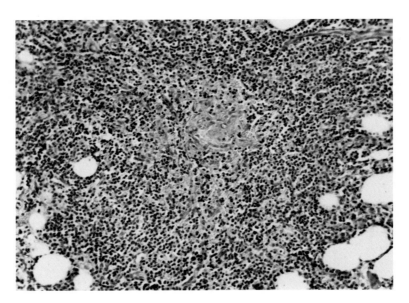

Figure 9-32
PAS-positive precipitate in bone marrow lymphoid nodules in monoclonal macroglobulinemia. (PAS, ×154.)

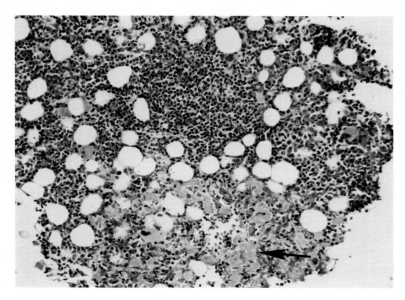

Figure 9-33
Hyaline precipitate (*arrow*), PAS positive, negative for amyloid, adjacent to lymphoid nodule in a patient with monoclonal macroglobulinemia. (H&E, ×154.)

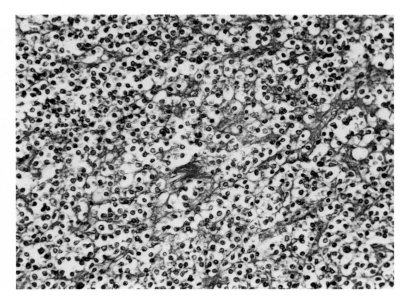

Figure 9-34
PAS-positive linear precipitates in lymphoid follicle of a patient with monoclonal macroglobulinemia. (PAS, ×308.)

References

1. Albahary, C., Ripault, J., Guillaume, J., Legrand, P., and Martin, S. La réticulose histiolymphocytaire avec myélofibrose. *Presse Med.* 35: 1531, 1970.
2. Aschoff, L. Das reticulo-endotheliale System. *Ergeb. Inn. Med. Kinderheilkd.* 26:1, 1924.
3. Aschoff, L., and Kiyono, K. Zur Frage der grossen Mononukleären. *Folia Haematol.* 15:383, 1913.
4. Askanazy, M. Uber die Lymphfollikel im menschlichen Knochenmark. *Virchows Arch. Pathol. Anat.* 220:257, 1915.
5. Baehr, G., and Klemperer, P. Giant follicle lymphoblastoma. *N.Y. State J. Med.* 40:7, 1940.
6. Catovsky, D., Petit, J. E., Galetto, J., Okos, A., and Galton, D. A. G. The B-lymphocyte nature of the hairy cell leukemic reticuloendotheliosis. *Br. J. Haematol.* 26:29, 1974.
7. Chomette, G., Dumont, J., Pinaudeau, Y., Auriol, M., and Brocheriou, C. Les îlots lymphoides dans la moëlle osseuse. *Ann. Anat. Pathol.* 12:91, 1967.
8. Duhamel, G. Les localisations à la moëlle osseuse des lymphosarcomes. *Ann. Anat. Pathol.* 9:197, 1964.
9. Duhamel, G. Les nodules lymphoides de la moëlle osseuse. *Presse Med.* 76:1947, 1968.
10. Duhamel, G. Lymphoid myelofibrosis: About 10 further observations. *Acta Haematol.* 45:89, 1971.
11. Ewing, J. Endothelioma of lymph nodes. *J. Med. Res.* 28:1, 1913.
12. von Fischer, O. Uber die Lymphknötchen im menschlichen Humerus-Wirbel und Rippenmarke. *Frankf. Z. Pathol.* 20:347, 1917.
13. Flandrin, G., Boiron, M., Lasneret, J., Ripault, J., Lortholary, P,, Tanzer, J., and Bernard, J. Etude par biopsie des infiltrations lymphocytaires de la moëlle osseuse. *Presse Med.* 75:2497, 1967.
14. Flandrin, G., Daniel, M. T., Foucarde, M., and Chelloul, N. Leucémie à "tricholeucocyte" (hairy cell leukemia): Etude clinique et cytologique de 55 observations. *Nouv. Rev. Fr. Hematol.* 13:609, 1973.
15. Flandrin, G., and Ripault, J. Histio-lymphocytose médullaire et splénique de l'adulte: Etude de 19 cas. *Actual. Hematol.* 3:18, 1969.
16. van Furth, R. Origin and kinetics of monocytes and macrophages. *Semin. Hematol.* 7:125, 1970.
17. Hansen, J. A., and Good, R. A. Malignant disease of the lymphoid system in immunological perspective. *Hum. Pathol.* 5:567, 1974.
18. Hashimoto, M., Masanori, H., and Tsukasa, S. Lymphoid nodules in human bone marrow. *Acta Pathol. Jap.* 7:33, 1957.
19. Jaffe, E. S., Shevach, E. M., Frank, M. M., and Green, I. Leukemic reticuloendotheliosis: Presence of a receptor for cytophilic antibody. *Am. J. Med.* 57:108, 1974.
20. Jaffe, E. S., Shevach, E. M., Frank, M. M., et al. Nodular lymphoma—evidence for origin from follicular B lymphocytes. *N. Engl. J. Med.* 290:813, 1974.
21. Johnstone, M. The appearance and significance of tissue mast cells in human bone marrow. *Am. J. Clin. Pathol.* 7:275, 1954.
22. Leder, L. D. Uber die selektive fermentcytochemische Darstellung von neutrophilen myeloischen Zellen und Gewebsmastzellen in Paraffinschnitt. *Klin. Wochenschr.* 42:533, 1964.

23. Lennert, K. *Pathologie der Halslymphknoten.* Berlin: Springer, 1964. P. 67.
24. Lennert, K. Follicular Lymphoma—A Tumor of the Germinal Centers. In K. Akazaki, H. Rappaport, C. W. Berard, J. M. Bennett, and E. Ishikawa (Eds.), *Malignant Diseases of the Hematopoietic System* (Gann Monograph on Cancer Research 15). Tokyo: University of Tokyo Press, 1973. Pp. 217–225.
25. Lennert, K., and Nagai, K. Quantitative und qualitative Gitterfaser-studien im Knochenmark: Normales Knochenmark. *Virchows Arch. Pathol. Anat.* 336:151, 1962.
26. Lennert, K., and Nagai, K. Quantitative und qualitative Gitterfaser-studien im Knochenmark: Chronische lymphatische Leukämie. *Virchows Arch. Pathol. Anat.* 340:25, 1965.
27. Levine, G. D., and Dorfman, R. F. Nodular lymphoma: An ultra-structural study of its relationship to germinal centers and a correlation of light and electron microscopic findings. *Cancer* 35:148, 1975.
28. Liao, K. T. The superiority of histologic sections of aspirated bone marrow in malignant lymphomas. *Cancer* 27:618, 1971.
29. Lukes, R. J., Butler, J. J., and Hicks, E. B. Natural history of Hodgkin's disease as related to its pathologic picture. *Cancer* 19:317, 1966.
30. Lukes, R. J., and Collins, R. D. New Observations on Malignant Lymphoma. In K. Akazaki, H. Rappaport, C. W. Berard, J. M. Bennett, and E. Ishikawa (Eds.), *Malignant Diseases of the Hematopoietic System* (Gann Monograph on Cancer Research 15). Tokyo: University of Tokyo Press, 1973. Pp. 209–215.
31. Lukes, R. J., Craver, L. F., Hall, T. C., et al. Report of the Nomen-clature Committee. *Cancer Res.* 26:1311, 1966.
32. Neiman, R. S., Rosen, P. J., and Lukes, R. J. Lymphocyte-depletion Hodgkin's disease: A clinicopathologic entity. *N. Engl. J. Med.* 288:751, 1973.
33. Oberling, C. Les réticulo-sarcomes et les réticulo-endothélio-sarcomes de la moëlle osseuse. *Bull. Assoc. Fr. Etud. Cancer* 17:259, 1928.
34. Pettet, J. D., Pease, G., and Cooper, T. An evaluation of paraffin sections of aspirated marrow in malignant lymphoma. *Blood* 10:820, 1955.
35. Rappaport, H. Tumors of the Hematopoietic System. In *Atlas of Tumor Pathology.* Washington, D.C.: Armed Forces Institute of Pathology, 1966. Sect. III, Fasc. 8, pp. 10, 28.
36. Rappaport, H., Winter, W. J., and Hicks, E. C. Follicular lymphoma—a reevaluation of its position in the scheme of malignant lymphoma based on a survey of 253 cases. *Cancer* 9:792, 1956.
37. Rohr, K. *Das menschliche Knochenmark.* Stuttgart: Thieme, 1960. Pp. 340, 467.
38. Roulet, R. Das primäre Retothelsarkom der Lymphknoten. *Virchows Arch. Pathol. Anat.* 277:15, 1930.
39. Rywlin, A. M., Ortega, R. S., and Dominguez, C. J. Lymphoid nodules of bone marrow: Normal and abnormal. *Blood* 43:389, 1974.
40. Rywlin, A. M., Civantos, F., Ortega, R. S., and Dominguez, C. J. Bone marrow histology in monoclonal macroglobulinemia. *Am. J. Clin. Pathol.* 63:769, 1975.
41. Seligman, M. Introduction et anomalies des immunoglobulines. *Actual. Hematol.* 2:63, 1968.

42. Waitz, R., Mayer, S., Bigel, P., and Fitzenkam-Saito, A. Myeloscleroses chroniques à forme lymphoide. *Nouv. Rev. Fr. Hematol.* 3:490, 1963.
43. Werner, W. Die Lymphknötchen im menschlichen Knochenmark. *Frankf. Z. Pathol.* 70:398, 1960.
44. Williams, R. J. The lymphoid nodules of human bone marrow. *Am. J. Clin. Pathol.* 15:377, 1939.
45. Yam, L. T., Li, C. Y., and Finkel, H. E. Leukemic reticulo-endotheliosis. *Arch. Intern. Med.* 130:248, 1972.

10 Foreign Cells

Metastatic Tumor Cells

Metastatic tumor cells are much easier to recognize and are found more frequently in histologic sections than in smears of aspirated bone marrow. Roeckel [30] has stated that bone marrow biopsy is superior to histologic sections of aspirated marrow in the diagnosis of metastatic malignancy. However, because technics for aspirating and processing marrow for preparation of histologic sections vary greatly, it is difficult to substantiate this view. We have attempted to establish a norm for comparing the efficiency of recovery of metastatic carcinoma by different modalities of clinical bone marrow sampling. Thus the incidence of metastatic carcinoma to the bone marrow in a series of 220 consecutive autopsies of patients with carcinoma was found to be 34.5 percent by routine autopsy technic. Histologic sections of bone marrow aspirates performed at autopsy by an identical method to that used in living patients revealed metastatic carcinoma in 10 percent of the patients, or somewhat less than a third of the cases in which metastases were demonstrable with routine autopsy technic [37] (see also Chap. 1). A comparative figure for the incidence of metastatic carcinoma when the marrow is sampled by needle biopsy is not available.

The vast majority of metastatic tumor cells observed in adult patients are derived from carcinomas and originate most frequently in the prostate, breast, or lung. However, carcinomas originating in other organs such as the stomach, thyroid, pancreas, or kidney may involve the bone marrow. Malignant melanomas may replace the bone marrow extensively. In children, neuroblastomas frequently metastasize to the bone marrow. Metastatic carcinoma cells are larger than nucleated red cells or the precursors of the granulocytic series and can be easily spotted under low power. Carcinoma cells occur in groups which may completely replace the hematopoietic and fat cells of the normal marrow (Fig. 10-1). Occasionally, there are preserved fat cells among the carcinoma cells (Fig. 10-2). When aspirated, the tumor cells often have a tendency to break away from the hematopoietic marrow (Figs. 10-3, 10-4). The carcinoma cells may be arranged in solid sheets (Fig. 10-4), in cords, i.e., in a trabecular pattern (see Fig. 10-2), or in a glandular pattern (Figs. 10-5, 10-6, 10-7). They may show a squamous pattern, i.e., exhibit intercellular bridges and/or keratinization (Figs. 10-8, 10-9). In general, the pattern of the metastatic tumor tends to resemble the primary neoplasm.

Metastatic carcinoma from the prostate may exhibit a glandular or a solid growth pattern (see Fig. 10-7; Fig. 10-10). The cells may have a vacuolated and granular appearance (Fig. 10-10). The vacuolated ap-

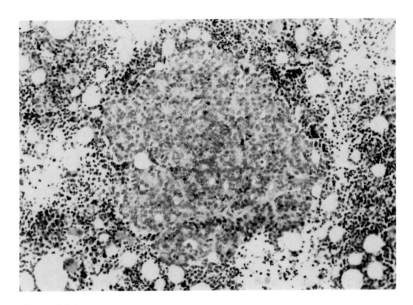

Figure 10-1
Solid island of carcinoma completely replacing hematopoietic and fatty marrow. (H&E, ×176.)

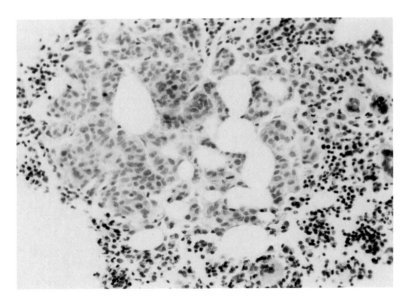

Figure 10-2
Trabecular arrangement of carcinoma cells with partial preservation of fat
cells. (H&E, ×354.)

134   10: Foreign Cells

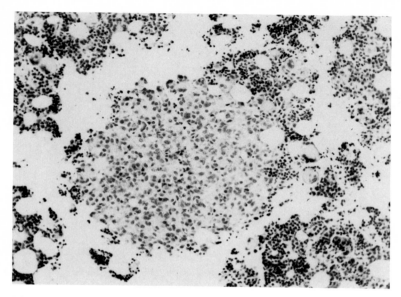

Figure 10-3
Solid island of carcinoma cells breaking away from hematopoietic elements.
(H&E, ×198.)

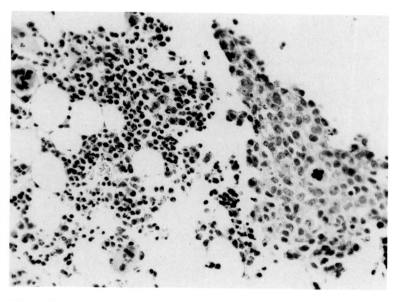

Figure 10-4
Solid sheet of carcinoma cells which have broken away from hematopoietic
elements. Note atypical mitotic figure. (H&E, ×374.)

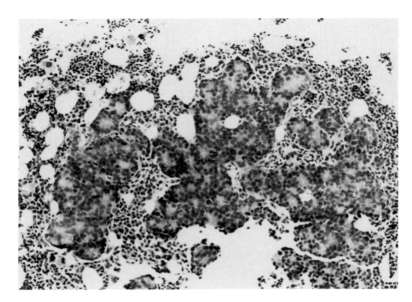

Figure 10-5
Metastatic adenocarcinoma. Note glandular arrangement of tumor cells.
(H&E, ×416.)

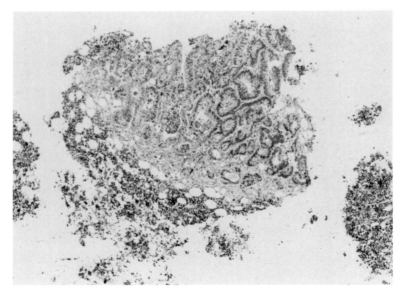

Figure 10-6
Metastatic adenocarcinoma. Glandular lumens are larger than in Figure 10-5.
(H&E, ×63.)

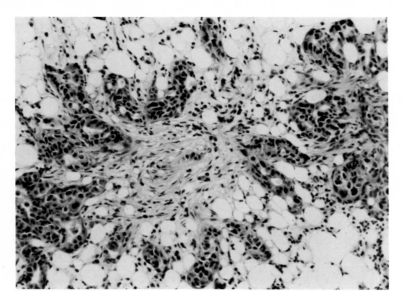

Figure 10-7
Prostatic adenocarcinoma metastatic to bone marrow. Note associated focal myelofibrosis. (H&E, ×134.)

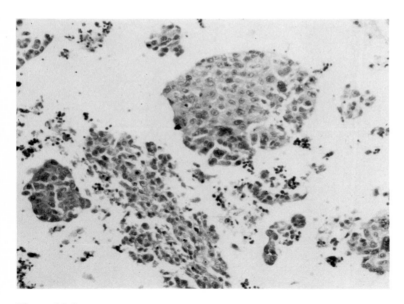

Figure 10-8
Bronchogenic squamous cell carcinoma metastatic to bone marrow. The carcinoma cells are arranged in solid sheets, which have broken away from the hematopoietic marrow. There is no keratinization. Intercellular bridges cannot be seen at this magnification. (H&E, ×162.)

137

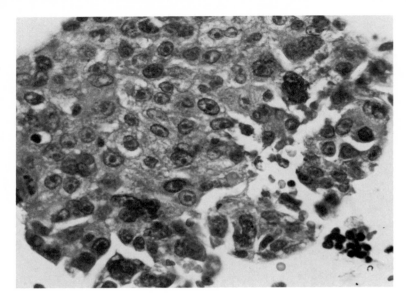

Figure 10-9
Metastatic bronchogenic squamous cell carcinoma. Note prominent nucleoli.
(H&E, ×430.)

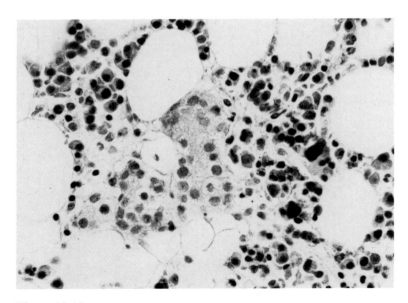

Figure 10-10
Metastatic carcinoma from prostate. Note foamy and granular appearance of
tumor cells. (H&E, ×565.)

pearance of the cytoplasm may be due to a high content of fat. Metastatic renal cell carcinoma may look very much like foam cells (Fig. 10-11). Variability in nuclear size, prominent nucleoli, and a tendency to gland formation help in the differential diagnosis. Also, cells from a metastatic renal cell carcinoma often contain glycogen in addition to fat. The glycogen can be demonstrated with a positive PAS stain which becomes negative if preceded by diastase digestion. Granular PAS-positive carcinoma cells can also be derived from other primary carcinomas including those of the pancreas and salivary glands.

Bronchogenic carcinomas, particularly of the undifferentiated small cell type (oat cell carcinoma), frequently metastasize to the bone marrow [12]. The cells of this tumor display relatively small nuclei, often somewhat elongated, with considerable variation in size and shape (Fig. 10-12). There is relatively little stroma separating the tumor cells.

We have seen a metastatic carcinoid tumor in the bone marrow of two patients. These tumor cells appear in solid sheets (Fig. 10-13). The cells are smaller and the nuclei are more regular than the usual carcinoma cells. They can be confused with reticulum cell sarcomas. An argentaffin stain may be helpful in confirming the diagnosis; however, not all carcinoids have argentaffin-positive granules in their cytoplasm.

Rarely a collision tumor can be seen in the bone marrow. Thus we have seen a carcinoma of the prostate associated with a multiple myeloma and an adenocarcinoma colliding with a malignant lymphoma (Fig. 10-14).

The bone and bone marrow adjacent to metastatic tumor deposits may react in different ways. They may be entirely normal. The marrow may be extensively replaced by fibrous tissue so that marrow aspiration may fail and a needle biopsy has to be performed. Metaplastic bone formation may be observed in the fibrous tissue and may be associated with new endosteal bone formation (see Fig. 11-1). This combination of metaplastic and endosteal new bone formation is the basis of osteosclerosis. Resorption of bone trabeculae leads to osteopenia, that is, inadequate numbers and thinner bone trabeculae. Osteosclerosis or osteopenia may characterize the radiologic findings. Histologically, both processes may be seen, though one often predominates. The pathogenic factors determining formation or resorption of bone in association with a neoplasm are not well understood.

The marrow surrounding metastatic tumor nodules may be hypercellular or hypocellular. The hypercellularity may involve megakaryocytes, the red cell series, and the granulocytic series. Occasionally, only megakaryocytes will be increased (see Fig. 4-20). A marked increase in eosinophils may be noted. In my experience, plasma cells are often increased in the presence of metastatic carcinoma of the prostate, perhaps due to associated chronic pyelonephritis.

The peripheral blood is often normal in the presence of bone marrow metastases. Unexplained anemia, thrombocytosis, or eosinophilia should always prompt a search for metastatic bone marrow lesions. Occasionally, the anemia is associated with a leukoerythroblastic peripheral

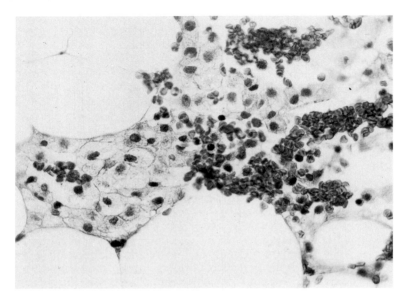

Figure 10-11
Metastatic renal cell carcinoma. Note resemblance of tumor cells to foam cells. Nuclei are larger than in histiocytic foam cells. The cytoplasm of renal cell carcinoma contains glycogen and is PAS positive. (H&E, ×565.)

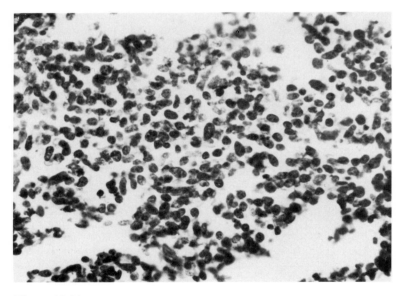

Figure 10-12
Bronchogenic oat cell carcinoma, metastatic to bone marrow. Note small, dark, somewhat elongated nuclei. (H&E, ×430.)

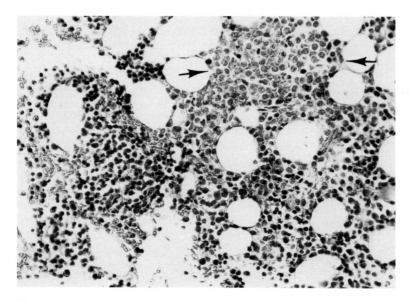

Figure 10-13
Carcinoid tumor metastatic to bone marrow. Tumor cells are arranged in solid sheets (*between arrows*). They are rather small and exhibit fairly regular nuclei. (H&E, ×374.)

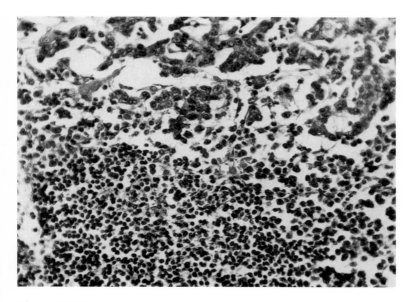

Figure 10-14
Collision tumor. Metastatic adenocarcinoma (*upper half*) and malignant lymphoma. (H&E, ×374.)

blood, that is, the presence of immature granulocytes and nucleated red blood cells. A syndrome characterized by severe hemolytic anemia with irregularly contracted red blood cells, thrombocytopenia, and fibrinogenopenia can be seen with carcinomas of the stomach, pancreas, breast, or lung. Metastases in this syndrome are often microscopic and associated with tumor thrombi in small vessels. In such instances the bone marrow and lung show the most extensive metastases [17]. The importance of the microangiopathy for the hemolytic anemia in this syndrome was stressed by Brain et al. [6]. This syndrome is an example of a consumption coagulopathy caused by disseminated intravascular coagulation.

Foam Cells

Foam cells occur in the bone marrow following fat necrosis due to trauma, pancreatitis, or infarction. These foam cells have a granular cytoplasm with fine, regular vacuoles and somewhat eccentrically placed nuclei. Often they are associated with microcysts resulting from the confluence of fat vacuoles after the breakdown of the plasma membranes of fat cells (Fig. 10-15). Foam cells are also known as xanthoma cells, pseudoxanthoma cells, and lipophages. They resemble metastatic renal cell carcinoma, but they do not have prominent nucleoli or cytoplasmic glycogen.

Foam cells can be seen in the bone marrow in a variety of diseases. Particularly prominent in Niemann-Pick disease, they are also present in other sphingolipidoses such as Fabry's disease, in eosinophilic granuloma, Hand-Schüller-Christian disease, and Tangier disease [2], in hyperlipoproteinemias, and in some mucolipidoses [35]. The diagnosis of the underlying disease responsible for the foam cells has to be based on other laboratory, clinical, and genetic studies. Histochemical studies have to be performed on smears or frozen sections of bone marrow because the embedding process removes most lipids. In the mucopolysaccharidoses, the bone marrow contains macrophages filled with metachromatic inclusions [7, 18]. These inclusions may also be encountered in plasma cells, lymphocytes, and granulocytes [7, 18]. Because these mucopolysaccharides are markedly water soluble, histologic sections of bone marrow fixed in formalin, an aqueous fixative, reveal vacuolated macrophages. Wolfe [42] has recommended that dioxane-fixed tissue be used for nonaqueous staining, and that prior to aqueous fixing or staining the acid mucopolysaccharides be rendered insoluble by precipitation with cetyltrimethylammonium bromide [42].

Occasionally the bone marrow contains an increased number of macrophages which give it a "starry-sky" appearance (Fig. 10-16). These macrophages appear under low magnification as round, empty spaces. Under higher magnification there is a faintly vacuolated cytoplasm with some granular debris and a peripherally located, small nucleus (Fig. 10-16).

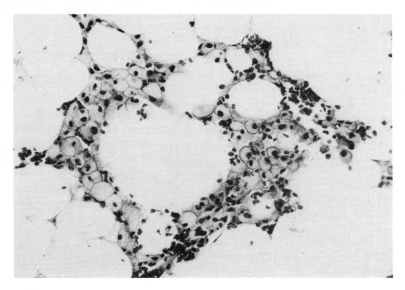

Figure 10-15
Foam cells in the bone marrow following fat necrosis caused by fracture. The foam cells are surrounding a microcyst. Note resemblance to metastatic renal cell carcinoma (see Fig. 10-11). (H&E, ×220.)

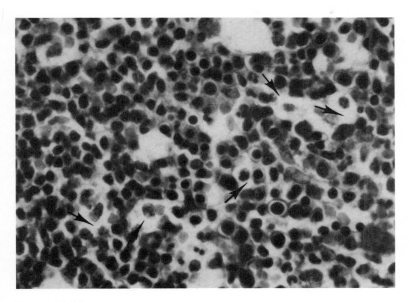

Figure 10-16
Increased number of bone marrow macrophages resulting in "starry-sky" appearance (*arrows*). The cytoplasm of the macrophages appears faintly vacuolated, almost empty. The nuclei, when hit by the plane of the section, are peripheral in position. (H&E, ×580.)

143

Ceroid-Containing Histiocytes (Sea-Blue Histiocytes, Blue Pigment Macrophages)

The unsaturated fatty acids contained in lipids of foamy macrophages may undergo peroxidation and polymerization to a pale yellow to dark brown pigment called ceroid [14]. The term *ceroid,* derived from the Greek and meaning "waxlike," was first introduced by Lillie et al. [24] to describe a pigment occurring in experimental dietary cirrhosis in rats. Lipofuscin and ceroid have the same histochemical characteristics. Because the exact chemical structure of these two compounds is unknown, it is uncertain whether they are identical. At present, *lipofuscin* is the preferred term for the naturally occurring age-related pigment, whereas *ceroid* is used for a similar pigment seen in different experimental and pathologic conditions. Ceroid may accumulate in neurones, muscle cells, epithelia, and histiocytes. Ceroid-containing histiocytes have been found in the bone marrow and spleen in a variety of conditions (see list below).

Conditions with Ceroid-containing Histiocytes in the Spleen and/or Bone Marrow

Batten's disease [20]
Niemann-Pick disease [8]
Tay-Sachs disease [20]
Adult lipidosis resembling Niemann-Pick disease [39]
Wolman's disease [25]
Ceroid accumulation in a patient with progressive neurologic disease [23]
Ceroid storage disease [27]
Chronic granulomatous disease of childhood [3]
Familial lipochrome histiocytosis [10]
Ceroid histiocytosis of spleen with rupture in a vegetarian [40]
Vascular pseudohemophilia associated with ceroid pigmentophagia in albinos [4, 15]
Hyperlipoproteinemia [29, 32]
Ceroid histiocytosis of spleen and bone marrow in ITP [31]
Syndrome of the sea-blue histiocyte (idiopathic ceroid histiocytosis of spleen and marrow)[a] [33, 38]
Chronic granulocytic leukemia[b] [36]
Sickle cell anemia[b] [19]
Cirrhosis of the liver[b] [26]
Familial lecithin : cholesterol acyl transferase deficiency [16]

[a] Only the first patient of Silverstein et al. was examined and shown to have ceroid-containing splenic histiocytes. Because the Giemsa reaction for ceroid is not specific, it is possible that in the other cases of this syndrome, the sea-blue histiocytes may contain a different pigment.

[b] These patients had sea-blue histiocytes in the bone marrow. Because the Giemsa stain is nonspecific for ceroid, the nature of the pigment is unproved.

Source: Modified from A. M. Rywlin, J. A. Hernandez, D. E. Chastain, and V. Pardo, Ceroid histiocytosis of spleen and bone marrow in idiopathic thrombocytopenic purpura (ITP): A contribution to the understanding of the sea-blue histiocyte. *Blood* 37:587–593, 1971. By permission of Grune & Stratton.

They may result from an excessive phagocytosis of unsaturated lipids and/or a congenital inadequacy to catabolize unsaturated lipids. It should be remembered that unsaturated lipids are ubiquitous in biologic material because they are a constituent of cellular membranes and of subcellular organelles. Ceroid can be formed whenever there is a supply of unsaturated lipids and oxidants or a lack of antioxidants. Its production has been studied in vivo and in vitro [13].

The histochemical reactions of ceroid vary and reflect its degree of oxidation and polymerization [14]. The sine qua non for the identification of ceroid is insolubility in hydrocarbon lipid solvents and reactivity with fat stains such as oil red O and Sudan black (Table 10-1). The other histochemical reactions develop as the pigment ages: golden yellow autofluorescence first, followed by diastase-resistant PAS positivity and finally acid-fastness [14]. With the Giemsa-Wright stain, ceroid granules stain sea-blue or navy blue [31, 32], which led in the past, before the recognition of the nature of the pigment, to the creation of terms such as *blue pigment macrophage* [26] and *sea-blue histiocyte* [33]. The Giemsa-Wright stain is not specific for ceroid and dyes other substances such as melanin, hemosiderin, and mast cell granules various shades of blue.

Ceroid-containing histiocytes appear in hematoxylin and eosin-stained sections as macrophages containing varying amounts of pale yellow to brown granules. Usually these are associated with some fat vacuoles (Fig. 10-17, Plate IV). Special stains confirm the ceroid nature of the pigment (see Table 10-1; Plate IV).

In 1970 Silverstein et al. [33] described a new entity, "the syndrome of the sea-blue histiocyte," characterized by a relatively benign course, splenomegaly, thrombocytopenia, and numerous sea-blue histiocytes in the bone marrow. Dr. Silverstein kindly permitted us to examine the

Table 10-1. Principal Staining Reactions of Ceroid

Stain	Reaction
Oil red O, frozen sections	+
Oil red O, Paraplast sections	+
Sudan black, frozen sections	+
Sudan black, Paraplast sections	+
Autofluorescense, frozen sections	Greenish yellow
Autofluorescense, Paraplast sections	Golden yellow
PAS	+
Diastase plus PAS	+
Peracetic acid–Schiff	+
Bromination plus peracetic acid–Schiff	—
Ziehl-Neelsen	Acid fast with age
Silver carbonate	Blackens slowly
Giemsa	Navy or sea blue

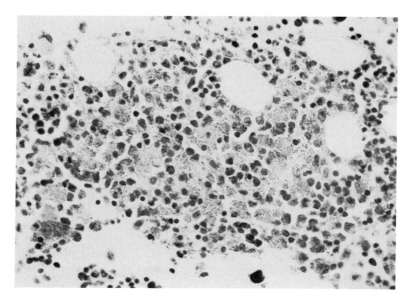

Figure 10-17
Ceroid-containing histiocytes. Note finely granular appearance of cytoplasm
(see also Plate IV). (H&E, ×600.)

spleen of his first case of the "sea-blue histiocyte syndrome" [34]. We
were able to show that the sea-blue granules in the histiocytes were
ceroid [31], and we have proposed that the syndrome be renamed
idiopathic ceroid histiocytosis of spleen and bone marrow [31, 38].
Prior to making this diagnosis, it is essential to eliminate all the entities
known to be associated with ceroid-containing histiocytes. This has not
been done in all cases of the syndrome of the sea-blue histiocyte. It
is particularly important that patients be investigated for lipoprotein
abnormalities, lecithin:cholesterol acyl transferase deficiency, and
sphingomyelinase deficiency. If sphingomyelinase deficiency is encountered, the patient's disorder should be classified in the Niemann-Pick
group of diseases.

Ceroid-containing histiocytes are often associated with increased
numbers of plasma cells. It is uncertain whether this is due to some
antigenic stimulation exerted by lipids or to the tendency of plasma cells
to aggregate around histiocytes (p. 78).

Gaucher's Cells

Gaucher's disease is characterized by a benign systemic proliferation of
histiocytes (reticulum cells, macrophages) whose cytoplasm is filled
with ceramide glucoside (cerebroglucoside). Ceramide glucoside is derived from the breakdown of a more complex substance (globoside)

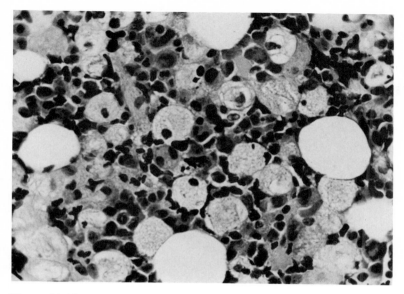

Figure 10-18
Numerous Gaucher's cells. Note granular, fibrillary, somewhat foamy cytoplasmic appearance. (H&E, ×494.)

which is found in the stroma of red blood cells and perhaps granulocytes. The reticuloendothelial cells, performing their function of phagocytosing senescent blood cells, are unable to catabolize globoside beyond the ceramide glucoside stage because they are deficient in a specific enzyme: beta glucosidase [5]. What triggers the proliferation of the histiocytes is not understood, but presumably it is a "reactive" process to the accumulated glucocerebroside. The proliferation of the histiocytes is responsible for the hepatosplenomegaly and characteristic bone changes in patients with Gaucher's disease.

Contrary to the foam cell of Niemann-Pick disease, the Gaucher's cell is almost pathognomonic for Gaucher's disease. It can be recognized easily in bone marrow sections and smears. In sections the cells are large, round to oval, and exhibit a relatively small, dark, eccentrically located nucleus (Fig. 10-18). The cytoplasm is granular but exhibits a faintly eosinophilic fibrillary pattern which is characteristic of the Gaucher's cell (Fig. 10-18) and which has been likened to wrinkled cigarette paper. Pure foam cells as well as histiocytes exhibiting vacuoles in addition to the characteristic fibrillary pattern are also present in Gaucher's disease. In histologic sections of Paraplast-embedded tissue, the Gaucher's cells display a moderate PAS positivity which is diastase resistant. Stains for hemosiderin give the cytoplasm a diffuse pale blue hue that is probably due to ferritin derived from ingested red blood cells [21]. Similar to ceroid histiocytes, Gaucher's cells may be associated

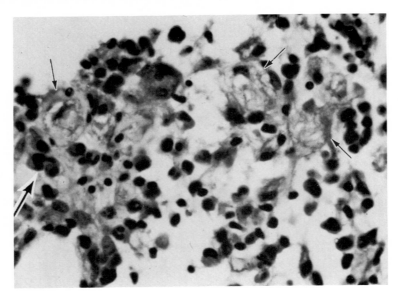

Figure 10-19
Typical Gaucher's cells (*thin arrows*) associated with plasma cells (*heavy arrow*). (H&E, ×267.)

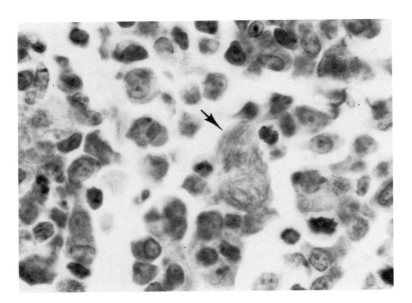

Figure 10-20
Gaucher-like cell in chronic granulocytic leukemia. Note almost crystalline cytoplasmic striations which are strongly PAS positive (*arrow*). (PAS, ×1050.)

with an increased number of plasma cells in the marrow (Fig. 10-19). This finding may explain the increased incidence of monoclonal gammopathies in Gaucher's disease [28].

Gaucher-like cells have been reported in chronic granulocytic leukemia [1], thalassemia [43], hereditary dyserythropoietic anemia [9], and rarely acute leukemia of childhood [41]. With the light microscope these cells appear identical with true Gaucher's cells (Fig. 10-20). However, based on electron microscopic studies, the identity and the distinctness of both Gaucher-like and true Gaucher's cells have been claimed [11, 22].

References

1. Albrecht, M. "Gaucher-Zellen" bei chronisch-myeloischer Leukämie. *Blut* 13:169, 1966.
2. Bale, P. M., Clifton-Bligh, P., Benjamin, B. N. P., and Whyte, H. M. Pathology of Tangier disease. *J. Clin. Pathol.* 24:609, 1971.
3. Bartman, J., Van der Velde, R. L., and Friedman, F. Pigmented lipid histiocytosis and susceptibility to infection: Ultrastructure of splenic histiocytes. *Pediatrics* 40:1000, 1967.
4. Bednar, B., Hermansky, F., and Lojda, Z. Vascular pseudohemophilia associated with ceroid pigmentophagia in albinos. *Am. J. Pathol.* 45:283, 1964.
5. Brady, R. O., Johnson, W. G., and Uhlendorf, B. W. Identification of heterozygous carriers of lipid storage diseases. *Am. J. Med.* 51:423, 1971.
6. Brain, M. C., Dacie, J. V., and Hourihane, O. B. Microangiopathic haemolytic anaemia: The possible role of vascular lesions in pathogenesis. *Br. J. Haematol.* 8:358, 1962.
7. Brunning, R. D. Morphologic alterations in nucleated blood and marrow cells in genetic disorders. *Hum. Pathol.* 1:99, 1970.
8. Crocker, A. C. Pigmentation in Lipidoses. In M. Wolman (Ed.), *Pigments in Pathology.* New York: Academic, 1969. P. 296.
9. Enquist, R. W., Gockerman, J. P., Jenis, E. H., Warkel, R. L., and Dillon, D. E. Type II congenital dyserythropoietic anemia. *Ann. Intern. Med.* 77:371, 1972.
10. Ford, D. K., Price, G. E., Culling, C. F. A., and Vassar, P. S. Familial lipochrome pigmentation of histiocytes with hyperglobulinemia, pulmonary infiltration, splenomegaly, arthritis and susceptibility to infection. *Am. J. Med.* 33:478, 1962.
11. Gerdes, J., Marathe, R. L., Bloodworth, J. M. B., and MacKinney, A. A. Gaucher cells in chronic granulocytic leukemia. *Arch. Pathol.* 88:194, 1969.
12. Hansen, H. H., Muggia, F. M., and Selawry, O. S. Bone-marrow examination in 100 consecutive patients with bronchogenic carcinoma. *Lancet* 2:443, 1971.
13. Hartroft, W. S., and Porta, E. A. In vitro and in vivo production of a ceroid-like substance from erythrocytes and certain lipids. *Science* 113:673, 1951.
14. Hartroft, W. S., and Porta, E. A. Ceroid. *Am. J. Med. Sci.* 250:324, 1965.

15. Hermansky, F., and Pudlak, P. Albinism associated with hemorrhagic diathesis and unusual pigmented reticular cells in the bone marrow: Report of two cases with histochemical studies. *Blood* 14:162, 1959.
16. Jacobsen, C. D., Gjone, E., and Hovig, T. Sea-blue histiocytes in familial lecithin:cholesterol acyl transferase deficiency. *Scand. J. Haematol.* 9:106, 1972.
17. Jarcho, S. Diffusely infiltrative carcinoma. *Arch. Pathol.* 22:674, 1936.
18. Jermain, L. F., Rohn, R. J., and Bond, W. H. Studies on the role of the reticuloendothelial system in Hurler's disease. *Am. J. Med. Sci.* 239:612, 1960.
19. Kattlove, H. E., Gaynor, E., Spivack, M., and Gottfried, E. L. Sea-blue indigestion. *N. Engl. J. Med.* 282:630, 1970.
20. Kristensson, K., and Sourander, P. Occurrence of lipofuscin in inherited metabolic disorders affecting the nervous system. *J. Neurol. Neurosurg. Psychiatry* 29:113, 1966.
21. Lee, R. E., Balcerzak, S. P., and Westerman, M. P. Gaucher's disease: A morphologic study and measurements of iron metabolism. *Am. J. Med.* 42:891, 1967.
22. Lee, R. E., and Ellis, L. D. The storage cells of chronic myelogenous leukemia. *Lab. Invest.* 24:261, 1971.
23. Levine, A. S., Lemieux, B., Brunning, R., White, J. G., Sharp, H. L., Stadlan, E., and Krivit, W. Ceroid accumulation in a patient with progressive neurological disease. *Pediatrics* 42:483, 1968.
24. Lillie, R. D., Ashburn, L. L., Sebrell, W. D., Daft, F. S., and Lowry, J. V. Histogenesis and repair of the hepatic cirrhosis in rats produced on low protein diets and preventable with choline. *Public Health Rep.* 57:502, 1942.
25. Lowden, J. A., Barson, A. J., and Wentworth, P. Wolman's disease: A microscopic and biochemical study showing accumulation of ceroid and esterified cholesterol. *Can. Med. Assoc. J.* 102:402, 1970.
26. Moeschlin, S. *Spleen Puncture.* New York: Grune & Stratton, 1951. Pp. 24, 55.
27. Oppenheimer, E. H., and Andrews, E. C. Ceroid storage disease in childhood. *Pediatrics* 23:1091, 1959.
28. Pratt, P. W., Estren, S., and Kochwa, S. Immunoglobulin abnormalities in Gaucher's disease: Report of 16 cases. *Blood* 31:633, 1968.
29. Roberts, W. C., Levy, R. I., and Fredrickson, D. S. Hyperlipoproteinemia: A review of the five types with first report of necropsy findings in type 3. *Arch. Pathol.* 90:46, 1970.
30. Roeckel, I. E. Diagnosis of metastatic carcinoma of bone marrow biopsy versus bone marrow aspiration. *Ann. Clin. Lab. Sci.* 4:193, 1974.
31. Rywlin, A. M., Hernandez, J. A., Chastain, D. E., and Pardo, V. Ceroid histiocytosis of spleen and bone marrow in idiopathic thrombocytopenia purpura (ITP): A contribution to the understanding of the sea-blue histiocyte. *Blood* 37:587, 1971.
32. Rywlin, A. M., Lopez-Gomez, A., Tachmes, P., and Pardo, V. Ceroid histiocytosis of the spleen in hyperlipemia: Relationship to the syndrome of the sea-blue histiocyte. *Am. J. Clin. Pathol.* 56:572, 1971.
33. Silverstein, M. N., Ellefson, R. D., and Ahern, E. F. The syndrome of the sea-blue histiocyte. *N. Engl. J. Med.* 282:1, 1970.
34. Silverstein, M. N., Young, D. G., Remine, W. H., and Pease, G. L. Splenomegaly with rare morphologically distinct histiocytes. *Arch. Intern. Med.* 114:251, 1964.

35. Spranger, J. W., and Wiedemann, H. R.   The genetic mucolipidoses: Diagnosis and differential diagnosis. *Humangenetik* 9:113, 1970.
36. Sundberg, R. A., Nelson, D. A., Hoilung, L. J., Herbst, G. H., and Beecher, N. B.   Cell-Debris and Blue Pigment Macrophages in Chronic Granulocytic Leukemia. Paper presented before the Tenth Congress of the International Society of Hematology, Stockholm, August–September, 1964.
37. Suprun, H., and Rywlin, A. M.   Metastatic carcinoma in histologic sections of aspirated bone marrow: A comparative autopsy study. *South. Med. J.* 69:438, 1976.
38. Teloh, H. A., and Rywlin, A. M.   Idiopathic ceroid histiocytosis of spleen: Syndrome of the sea-blue histiocyte. *Ann. Clin. Lab. Sci.* 2:175, 1972.
39. Terry, R. D., Sperry, W. M., and Brodoff, B.   Adult lipidosis resembling Niemann-Pick's disease. *Am. J. Pathol.* 30:263, 1954.
40. Winkler, H. H., Frame, B., Saeed, S. M., Spindler, A. C., and Brouillette, J. N.   Ceroid storage disease complicated by rupture of spleen. *Am. J. Med.* 46:297, 1969.
41. Witzleben, C. L., Drake, W. L., Jr., Sammon, J., and Mohabbat, O. M.   Gaucher's cells in acute leukemia of childhood. *J. Pediatr.* 76:129, 1970.
42. Wolfe, H. J.   Techniques for the histochemical localization of extremely water soluble acid mucopolysaccharides. *J. Histochem. Cytochem.* 12:217, 1964.
43. Zaino, E. C., Rossi, M. B., Pham, T. D., and Azar, H. A.   Gaucher's cells in thalassemia. *Blood* 38:457, 1971.

Collaborative Radiological Health Lab
Foothills Campus
Colorado State University
Fort Collins, Colorado 80523

11 Stromal Reactions

Myelofibrosis and Osteosclerosis

Myelofibrosis is best defined as replacement of the fatty and/or hemato-poietic tissue of bone marrow by fibrous tissue, that is, a tissue made up of fibroblasts and collagen fibers. The terms *myeloreticulosis* and *myelo-sclerosis* have been used as synonyms for myelofibrosis. Myeloreticulosis [10] refers to the increase in reticulin fibers, which are thin collagen fibers not visible in the hematoxylin and eosin stain but easily demonstrable by silver impregnations (see Appendix, 3). The term *reticulosis* is con-fusing in this connection because it is also used to describe proliferation of reticulum cells. Perhaps it is best to think of an increase in the reticulin fibers of the bone marrow as early myelofibrosis and refer to it as *reticulin myelofibrosis*. *Sclerosis* literally means "hardening," but the term is used by histologists also to describe a form of fibrosis consisting of thick, somewhat confluent collagen fibers in the presence of relatively few fibroblasts. Sclerosis represents a later stage of fibrosis in which the

Myelofibrosis

Bone diseases
   Osteitis fibrosa
   Renal osteodystrophy
   Paget's disease
   Fibrous dysplasia
   Osteopetrosis
   Fractures
Metastatic carcinoma
Inflammations
   Osteomyelitis
   Fat necrosis of marrow
   Late radiation myelitis
   Chemotherapy
Hematopoietic disorders
   Agnogenic myeloid metaplasia
   Polycythemia vera
   Refractory sideroblastic anemias
   Lymphoid myelofibrosis (hairy cell leukemia, leukemic reticuloendo-
      theliosis)
   Chronic lymphocytic leukemia
   Malignant myelosclerosis
   Familial myelofibrosis [9]

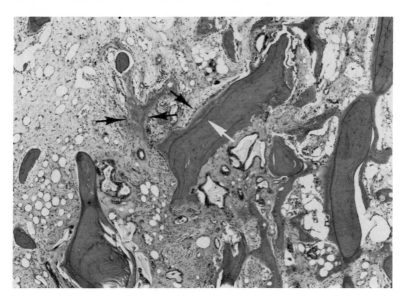

Figure 11-1
Myelofibrosis and osteosclerosis in metastatic adenocarcinoma. Note focus of metaplastic bone (*between paired left arrows*) and new endosteal bone formation (*upper black arrow*) separated from older trabecular bone by heavy cementing line (*white arrow*). (H&E, ×61.)

collagen fibers may appear as a confluent, eosinophilic, nonfibrillary material also called *hyaline fibrosis*. The collagenous nature of the material is apparent on electron microscopic examination. Not all eosinophilic hyaline-appearing materials are collagen. Some hyaline deposits react with special stains and can then be classified as amyloid, paramyloid, other protein deposits, or fibrinoid. Fibrinoid deposits have a more granular appearance.

Myelofibrosis may be associated with new bone formation, that is, osteosclerosis. The new bone may be lamellar or mature bone deposited on the endosteal surface of existing bone trabeculae (Fig. 11-1). It may also be immature bone (metaplastic, coarsely woven, fiberbone), which does not show the regular, parallel arrangement of collagen fibers seen in mature (lamellar) bone. This is particularly well brought out by viewing the bone with polarized light (see Fig. 12-1). Also, immature bone contains more and larger osteocytes (Chap. 12).

Myelofibrosis may be diffuse or localized, and it can be seen in many different diseases (see list on p. 153). The term should not be used as a synonym for agnogenic myeloid metaplasia, a fairly well defined myeloproliferative disorder associated with myelofibrosis and osteosclerosis. Myelofibrosis related to bone diseases and inflammations is rarely severe enough to produce hematologic abnormalities. Examples of this type of myelofibrosis are illustrated in Figures 1-6 to 1-8 and 12-7 to 12-9. Metastatic carcinoma to the bone marrow with extensive myelofibrosis may be associated with spenomegaly and extramedullary hematopoiesis.

In agnogenic myeloid metaplasia and in polycythemia vera there is a close association between reticulin and collagen fibers and megakaryocytes (see Figs. 4-16, 4-17). The increase in reticulin fibers in lymphoproliferative disorders is discussed and illustrated in Chapter 9. Lymphoid myelofibrosis is a synonym for hairy cell leukemia (see Fig. 9-31).

Malignant Myelosclerosis

Malignant myelosclerosis, first described by Lewis and Szur [3], appears to be a variant of an acute myeloblastic leukemia. The patients present with rapidly progressing anemia, thrombocytopenia, and leukopenia. The spleen is not palpable or may be moderately enlarged. A few blasts and nucleated red cells are noted in the peripheral blood. Bone marrow aspirations yield very few or no particles. Bone marrow biopsy shows extensive fibrosis, some megakaryocytes, and diffuse infiltration by immature cells probably representing myeloblasts (Fig. 11-2). Lubin et al. [6] reviewed the literature and reported three additional cases of this entity. They concluded that malignant myelosclerosis is best interpreted as an acute myeloproliferative disorder sharing features with acute leukemia and agnogenic myeloid metaplasia.

Serous Atrophy of Fat

In patients who have lost considerable weight the bone marrow fat exhibits characteristic changes. The fat cells become smaller and the spaces between them are filled with a faintly eosinophilic material representing serum and containing varying amounts of fibrin. This change is referred to as gelatinous or serous atrophy of fat (Figs. 11-3, 11-4). In cachectic individuals, the changes in the fat cells may be more severe: the single fat vacuole seen in normal adipocytes breaks up into several vacuoles of varying sizes (Fig. 11-5).

Fat Necrosis

Fat necrosis is observed in infarcts, fracture sites, and pancreatitis. Necrotic fat cells are invaded by macrophages which surround the fat vacuole and become lipophages or foam cells, that is, their cytoplasm is filled with many small, equal-sized vacuoles (Fig. 11-6). Necrotic fat cells may fuse, forming small cysts lined by foam cells (Fig. 11-7). These foam cells have been misinterpreted as lipoblasts and the fat necrosis was thought to represent regenerating fat tissue [1]. Such microcysts can also be seen in certain lipid granulomas, particularly in association with hyperlipoproteinemia (Fig. 11-8).

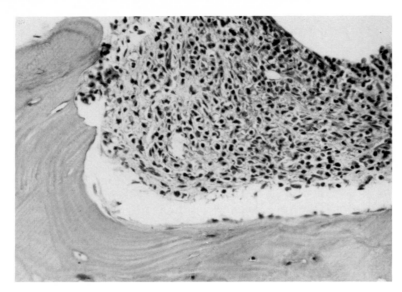

Figure 11-2
Malignant myelosclerosis. Hypercellular marrow and disappearance of fat cells. At this magnification the marrow resembles hairy cell leukemia (lymphoid myelofibrosis). However, at a higher power and with the Giemsa stain the blastic nature of the cells can be ascertained. Also note the lamellar appearance of the mature bone. (H&E, ×352.)

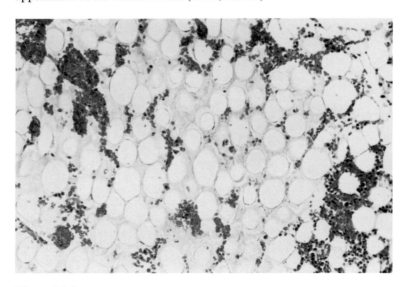

Figure 11-3
Serous atrophy of bone marrow fat. Fat cells are separated by protein-rich edema fluid. (H&E, ×176.)

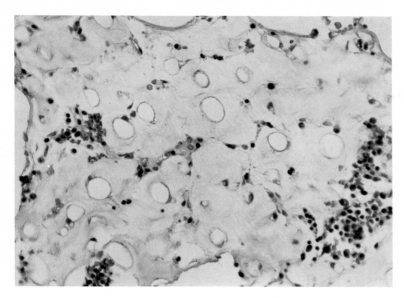

Figure 11-4
More advanced form of serous atrophy of fat. Only sparse hematopoietic
elements persist, and plasma cells appear increased. (H&E, ×352.)

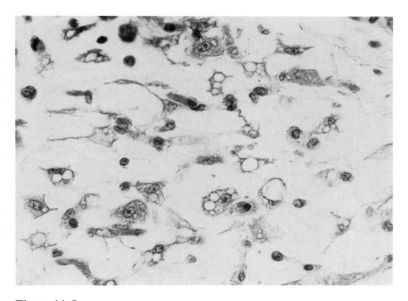

Figure 11-5
Atrophy of fat cells in severe cachexia. The single vacuole seen in normal
adipocytes is replaced by several vacuoles of varying size. (H&E, ×617.)

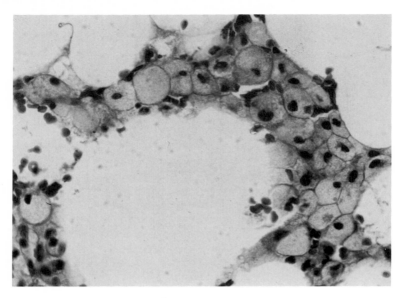

Figure 11-6
Foam cells in traumatic (fracture) fat necrosis. (H&E, ×565.)

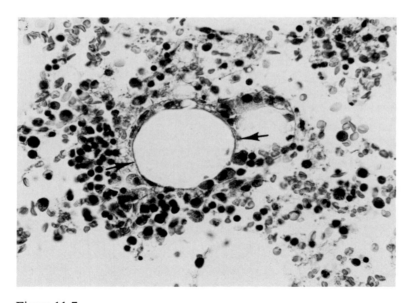

Figure 11-7
Microcystic fat necrosis (*small cyst between arrows*). Foam cells are seen in upper half of cyst wall lining. (H&E, ×617.)

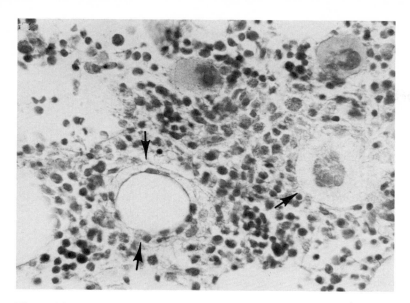

Figure 11-8
Microcystic lipid granuloma (*between arrows*) and Touton giant cell with characteristic peripherally vacuolated cytoplasm (*arrow*) in a juvenile diabetic with type IV hyperlipoproteinemia. (H&E, ×635.)

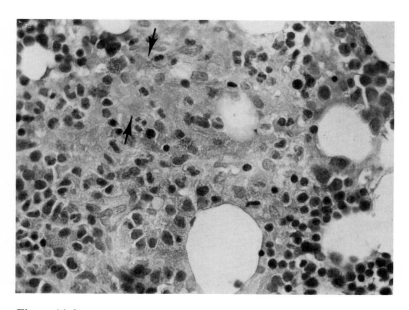

Figure 11-9
Small marrow hemorrhage. Note laked red blood cells (*arrows*). (H&E, ×565.)

Marrow Hemorrhage and Siderofibrotic Nodules

Acute marrow hemorrhage is difficult to diagnose with certainty because extravasation of red blood cells is produced during aspiration of the marrow. We diagnose marrow hemorrhage if the extravasated red blood cells show evidence of laking or sludging (Fig. 11-9). The sludged red cells have to be located inside of marrow particles, in the septa separating fat cells. Laking and sludging of red blood cells can be used as a criterion of in vivo extravasation of red cells only if formaldehyde or some other fixative is used that does not cause laking of red cells. In some hypocellular marrows there is an excess of red blood cells with relatively few nucleated hematopoietic cells (see Fig. 3-4). In the absence of sludging this should not be interpreted as hemorrhage. More extensive marrow hemorrhage is associated with disruption of fat cells and fat necrosis.

Occasionally, we have found small nodules in the marrow made up of fibroblasts and hemosiderin-containing macrophages. These siderofibrotic nodules resemble the Gandy-Gamna nodules of the spleen and probably represent organized small hemorrhages or old lipid granulomas (Fig. 11-10).

Acute Inflammation

Because the bone marrow normally contains many mature polymorphonuclear leukocytes, acute myelitis cannot be readily recognized. We have made this diagnosis in the presence of focal exudation of fibrin infiltrated predominantly by polymorphonuclear leukocytes (Fig. 11-11). If the exudation of fibrin is not accompanied by a significant cellular infiltrate, the lesion is referred to as *fibrinous myelitis* (Fig. 11-12). It is seen in patients receiving chemotherapy or irradiation. Fibrinous myelitis differs from serous atrophy of fat by the absence of atrophic fat cells. Also, the exudate is richer in fibrin.

Chronic Inflammation

In nonspecific chronic myelitis the normal marrow elements are replaced by a fibrinous exudate containing mast cells, plasma cells, lymphocytes, and a few polymorphonuclear leukocytes (Fig. 11-13). Such lesions can be seen in association with chemotherapy, radiation therapy, and systemic inflammatory diseases (Figs. 11-14, 11-15).

Granulomas

Granulomatous inflammation represents the reaction of the reticuloendothelial system to injury, and is characterized by the accumulation of histiocytes. Histiocytes are called *epithelioid cells* when they resemble epithelial cells by exhibiting a fairly abundant eosinophilic cytoplasm and appearing to touch each other. The histiocytes may be aggregated

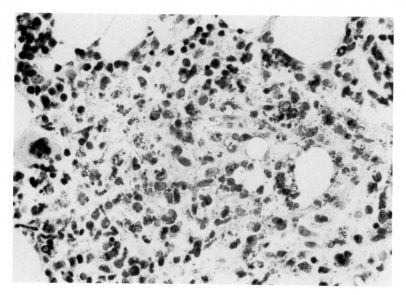

Figure 11-10
Siderofibrotic nodule. The granular material is hemosiderin. (H&E, ×617.)

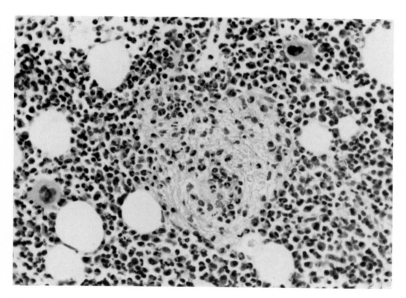

Figure 11-11
Focal acute myelitis. Exudation of fibrin infiltrated by polymorphonuclear leukocytes. (H&E, ×352.)

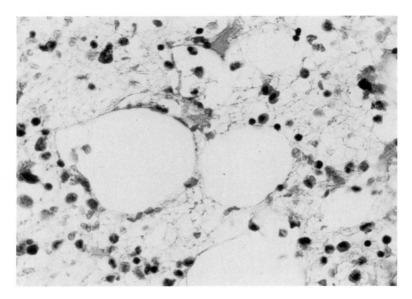

Figure 11-12
Fibrinous myelitis. Spaces separating fat cells are filled with fibrin displaying a characteristic fibrillary appearance. Only a few hematopoietic elements persist. Patient was receiving chemotherapy. (H&E, ×565.)

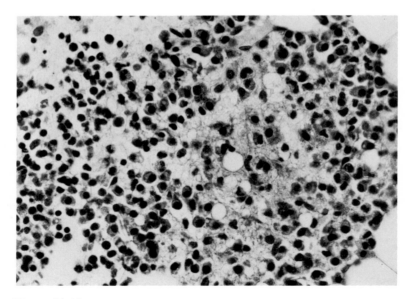

Figure 11-13
Focal, chronic, nonspecific myelitis. Normal marrow elements are replaced by fibrin, lymphocytes, and plasma cells. (H&E, ×565.)

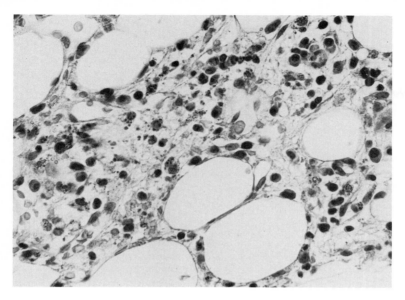

Figure 11-14
Fibrinous myelitis after chemotherapy. Note replacement of marrow elements by fibrin, hemosiderin-containing macrophages, and plasma cells. (H&E, ×617.)

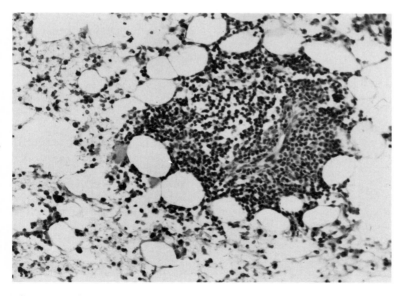

Figure 11-15
Fibrinous myelitis after radiation therapy. Note persistence of normal lymphoid follicle. (H&E, ×185.)

163

into fairly discrete nodules called *tubercles* or *granulomas*. These may be purely productive (without necrosis), or they may exhibit central necrosis (necrotizing or caseating granulomas) or suppuration (suppurative granulomas). Productive granulomas are characteristic, though not diagnostic, for sarcoidosis; necrotizing granulomas are seen in tuberculosis; and suppurative granulomas are seen in fungal diseases, tularemia, lymphopathia venereum, *Yersinia enterocolitica* infections, cat-scratch disease, and melioidosis.

Diffuse infiltration of a tissue by histiocytes without the formation of discrete nodules is called by some pathologists a diffuse granulomatous inflammation. Others use the term *granulomatous inflammation* only for instances in which histiocytes are aggregated into fairly discrete nodules (tuberculoid inflammation).

Lipid Granulomas

The most frequent granuloma encountered in bone marrow aspirates is the lipid granuloma. Lipid granulomas in the bone marrow are identical with those seen in the liver, spleen, and lymph nodes. We have encountered them in 9 percent of bone marrows [13]. They consist of a collection of macrophages containing fat vacuoles of various sizes, almost always smaller than the single vacuole in normal fat cells (Fig. 11-16). In addition to macrophages, lipid granulomas contain plasma cells, lymphocytes, a few eosinophils, and mast cells. Giant cells are present in 5 percent of lipid granulomas (Fig. 11-17). Well-formed foam cells are not present in the common type of lipid granuloma. Microcysts are seen occasionally; they are lined by compressed macrophages resembling the foam cells seen in fat necrosis (Fig. 11-18).

Some lipid granulomas show a finely granular, black, Prussian blue-negative pigment (Fig. 11-19). It is not formalin pigment, because it does not show double refractility and is not removed by an alcoholic solution of ammonium hydroxide. It probably represents anthracotic pigment. Occasionally, lipid granulomas are very rich in hemosiderin. Lipid granulomas exhibit an increased number of reticulin fibers (Fig. 11-20).

Lipid granulomas measure from 0.2 to 0.8 mm in greatest dimension and are usually located within or close to a lymphoid nodule or adjacent to a sinusoid (Fig. 11-21). With our technic of processing aspirated bone marrow particles, the number of lipid granulomas, when present, varies from 1 to 8 per slide. In some lipid granulomas, probably the older ones, fat vacuoles become less prominent and epithelioid cells appear (Figs. 11-22, 11-23). Occasionally, asteroid bodies can be found in the giant cells (Fig. 11-24). It is important to recognize this sarcoidlike appearance of some lipid granulomas in order to avoid making a diagnosis of a more serious granulomatous disease. By careful examination, macrophages with lipid vacuoles can always be found in sarcoidlike lipid granulomas. Furthermore, more characteristic lipid granulomas are found in association with sarcoidlike lipid granulomas.

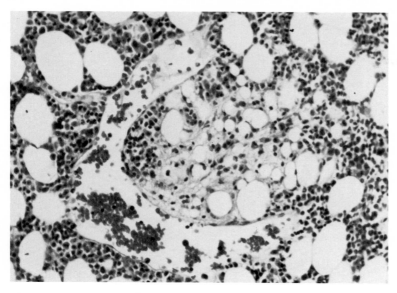

Figure 11-16
Lipid granuloma. Note relation to sinusoid and fat vacuoles, which vary
in size and are smaller than those in the normal fat cells. (H&E, ×222.)

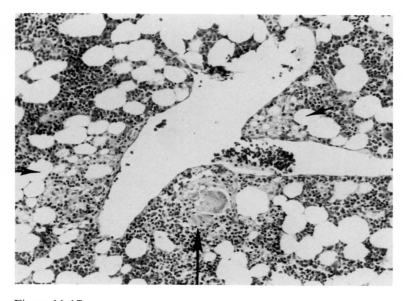

Figure 11-17
Lipid granulomas (*arrows*). Note relation to sinusoid and presence of giant
cells (*longer arrow*). (H&E, ×165.)

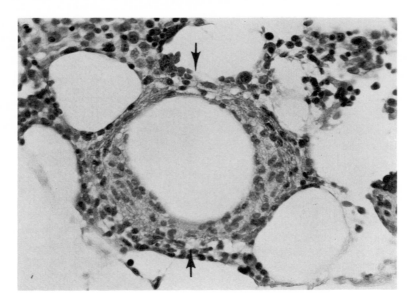

Figure 11-18
Lipid granuloma. Microcyst (*arrows*) lined by compressed histiocytes. (H&E,
×284.)

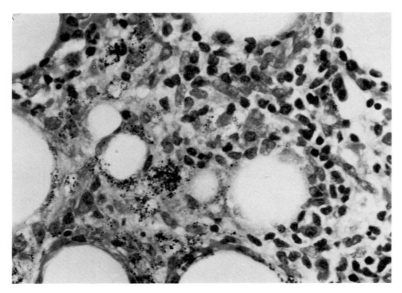

Figure 11-19
Lipid granuloma. Black, probably anthracotic, pigment. (H&E, ×441.)

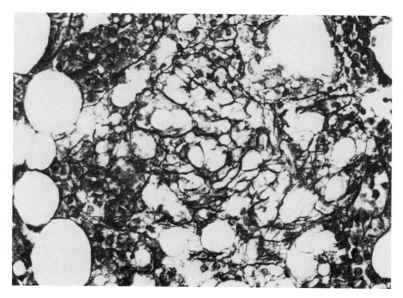

Figure 11-20
Lipid granuloma. Increased number of reticulin fibers. (Gordon-Sweets', ×220.)

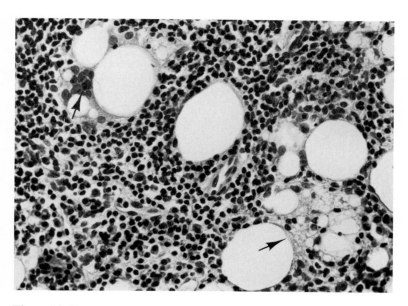

Figure 11-21
Lipid granulomas inside lymphoid follicle. Note giant cell (*arrow top left*) and microcyst formation (*arrow bottom right*). (H&E, ×330.)

167

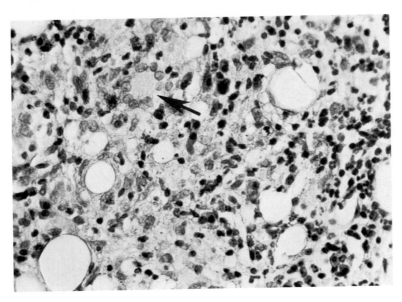

Figure 11-22
Aging lipid granuloma: fat vacuoles less prominent, giant cell (*arrow*), and epithelioid cells. (H&E, ×274.)

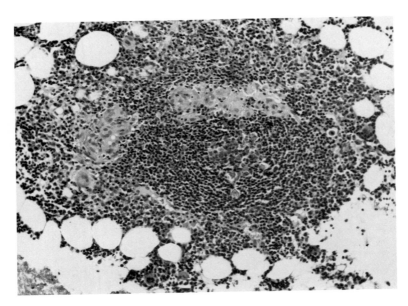

Figure 11-23
Sarcoidlike lipid granulomas composed of epithelioid cells within a lymphoid follicle. (H&E, ×198.)

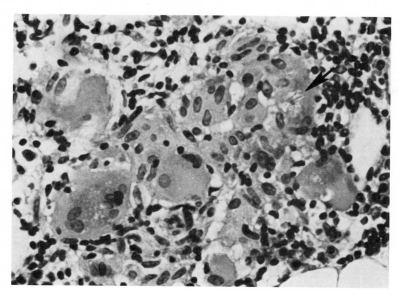

Figure 11-24
Sarcoidlike lipid granuloma containing giant cells and an asteroid body (*arrow*). (H&E, ×250.)

Lipid granulomas differ from serous atrophy of fat and from fat necrosis. In serous atrophy, the fat cells are smaller than normal and are separated by spaces filled with serous fluid and fibrin (see Fig. 11-3). Fat necrosis is characterized by the presence of fully developed foam cells and the formation of cysts (see Fig. 11-6).

Lipid granulomas do not seem to have any clinical significance. A somewhat higher incidence of diabetes and weight loss and higher average age were reported in patients with lipid granulomas [13].

The etiology and pathogenesis of lipid granulomas are unknown. Hudson and Robertson [2] have submitted suggestive evidence, by infrared spectrophotometry and thin-layer chromatography, that splenic lipid granulomas contain mineral oil. The morphologic appearance of lipid granulomas of the bone marrow is consistent with a reaction to mineral oil.

A different type of lipid granuloma can be seen in patients with hyperlipidemia. It consists of a collection of foam cells which may be associated with Touton-type giant cells (see Fig. 11-8). Ceroid-containing histiocytes have also been reported in hyperlipidemias [12] (see also Chap. 10).

Other Granulomas

Histologic sections of aspirated bone marrow particles often display granulomas in systemic granulomatous diseases. The study of such sections may contribute to the elucidation of a fever of unknown cause. We

169

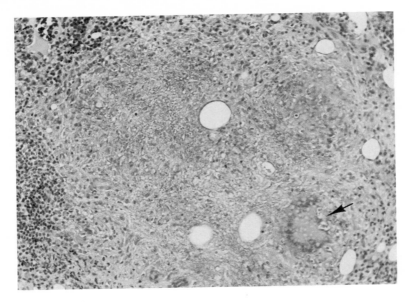

Figure 11-25
Caseating granuloma in miliary tuberculosis. Langhans' giant cell (*arrow*).
Acid-fast bacilli were demonstrated with Ziehl-Neelsen stain. (H&E, ×110.)

have observed specific granulomas in the marrow of patients with sarcoidosis and with miliary tuberculosis (Fig. 11-25). The frequency of marrow involvement in sarcoidosis is unknown. It is advisable to study histologic sections of aspirated bone marrow in patients suspected of having sarcoidosis prior to performing liver biopsy, a more dangerous and more costly procedure than bone marrow aspiration.

In one of our patients, a diagnosis of leprosy was established on histologic sections of a bone marrow aspirate (Fig. 11-26). Specific granulomas can also be seen in fungal diseases. Figure 11-27 demonstrates a granuloma in a patient with torulosis. In histoplasmosis numerous histiocytes filled with organisms are seen. The presence of a paranuclear body (kinetoplast) aids in differentiating leishmaniasis from histoplasmosis. Also, the PAS reaction stains the organisms causing histoplasmosis but does not stain leishmania. We have observed nonspecific granulomas in the bone marrow in typhoid fever, infectious mononucleosis, and viral hepatitis (Figs. 11-28 to 11-30). They have also been reported in brucellosis, glanders, and other diseases [10].

Sarcoidlike granulomas can be seen in the marrow of patients with Hodgkin's disease (Fig. 11-31). They should not be interpreted as evidence of marrow involvement by Hodgkin's disease.

We have also observed granulomatous myelitis of unknown etiology and pathogenesis (Fig. 11-32). Further studies are indicated to eluci-

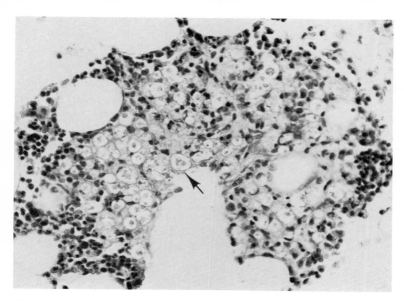

Figure 11-26
Lepromatous leprosy of bone marrow. Granuloma made up of Virchow cells: macrophages containing globi of acid-fast bacilli (*arrow*). A Fite stain is necessary to show that the globi contain acid-fast organisms. (H&E, ×220.)

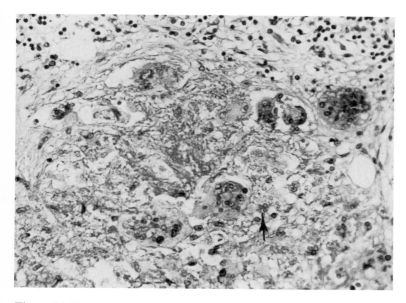

Figure 11-27
Cryptococcal granuloma. Note giant cells and budding yeast cells (*arrow*). (PAS, ×220.)

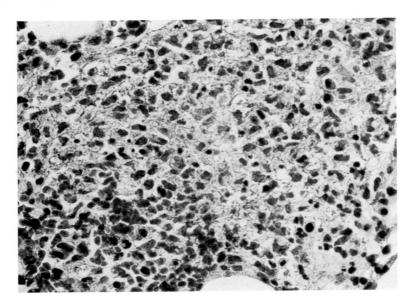

Figure 11-28
Poorly circumscribed granuloma in a patient with typhoid fever. Note epithelioid appearance of histiocytes. (H&E, ×494.)

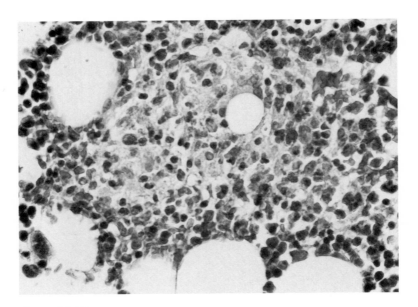

Figure 11-29
Small, nonspecific granuloma in a patient with infectious mononucleosis. (H&E, ×635.)

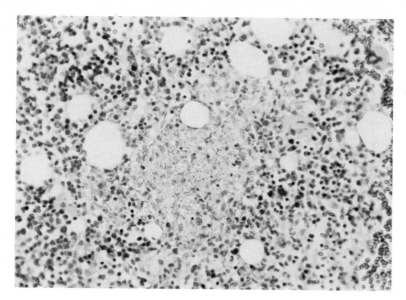

Figure 11-30
Focal granulomatous myelitis in a patient with viral hepatitis. Note fibrinous exudate and histiocytes. (H&E, ×384.)

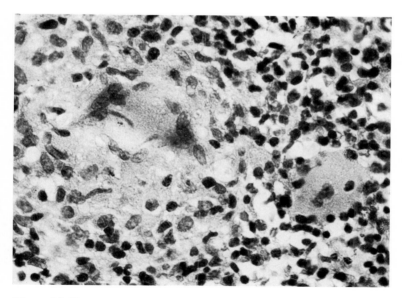

Figure 11-31
Sarcoidlike granuloma in a patient with Hodgkin's disease. (H&E, ×494.)

173

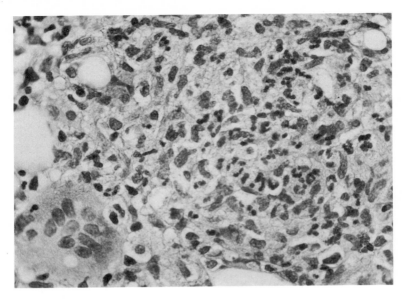

Figure 11-32
Granuloma with central collection of polymorphonuclear leukocytes (suppurative granuloma) of unknown etiology. (H&E, ×494.)

date the significance of such granulomas. Granulomatous myelitis can be caused by drugs (see below).

Eosinophilic Fibrohistiocytic Lesion
The eosinophilic fibrohistiocytic lesion represents a distinctive finding in the bone marrow, probably related to drug hypersensitivity [11]. The lesion consists of collections of cells characterized by regular, oval to spindle-shaped nuclei measuring 12 to 14 μ in length and 4 to 6 μ in width. These cells have an indistinct, amphophilic cytoplasm. They have been interpreted as histiocytes changing into fibroblasts. Among the fibrohistiocytes, there are numerous eosinophils, frequently forming dense aggregates, so-called eosinophilic abscesses. Some plasma cells and occasional mast cells are also present. This lesion cannot be identified in bone marrow smears.

On the basis of localization of the lesion, three types can be distinguished.

Type I is associated with lymphoid nodules (Figs. 11-33, 11-34; Plate IIIC, D). In this type, the fibrohistiocytes surround a central core of lymphocytes in a mantlelike fashion. In other instances of type I lesions, the fibrohistiocytes are located centrally inside a lymphoid nodule and are surrounded by lymphocytes. In still another variant of this lesions, the fibrohistiocytes are located centrally inside a lymphoid nodules and replace a segment of the lymphoid nodules.

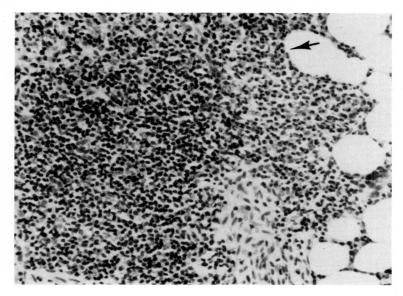

Figure 11-33
Eosinophilic fibrohistiocytic lesion, type I. Note lymphoid nodule with fibrohistiocytes at lower right corner. Collection of eosinophils which cannot be
recognized at this magnification (*arrow*). (H&E, ×153.)

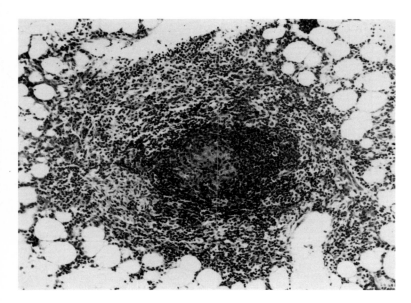

Figure 11-34
Eosinophilic fibrohistiocytic lesion, type I. Central lymphoid nodule with
hyaline deposit surrounded by histiocytes (see also Plate IIIC, D). (H&E,
×110.)

175

Type II is perivascular (Fig. 11-35). In a longitudinal section the lesion appears elongated and crescent-shaped and shows several oblique sections of a centrally placed vessel. No necrosis of vascular walls or thrombosis is present.

Type III is perisinusoidal and segmental (Fig. 11-36). This lesion is cap-shaped and is in close proximity to a segment of the wall of a bone marrow sinusoid.

All three types of lesions are cytologically identical. All the five patients in whom this lesion was reported showed lymphofollicular (type I) lesions. Perivascular (type II) lesions were present in four, and perisinusoidal lesions in two patients [11]. Hodgkin's disease, eosinophilic granuloma, Kaposi's sarcoma, and lipid granulomas have to be considered in the differential diagnosis. No Reed-Sternberg cells are present in these lesions. The regular, spindle-shaped appearance of the fibrohistiocytes and their lymphofollicular, perivascular, and perisinusoidal location rule out eosinophilic granuloma. The spindle cells in Kaposi's sarcoma are larger, and extravasated red blood cells can be seen among them. Lipid granulomas share with the eosinophilic fibrohistiocytic lesion the association with lymphoid nodules and sinusoids. Their appearance, however, is quite different (see p. 164).

The drugs apparently responsible for this lesion were ampicillin, allopurinol, and procainamide. In three patients in whom repeat bone marrows were available one month after the suspected drug had been discontinued, the fibrohistiocytic lesions could not be found [11].

Granulomatous Inflammation Probably Related to Drugs

We have observed in four patients a hitherto undescribed lesion which appears drug related. One of the patients was taking Diabinese, another allopurinol, and the remaining two procainamide. The bone marrow lesions consisted of numerous poorly circumscribed, partially confluent nodules made up of histiocytes and lymphocytes admixed with varying numbers of eosinophils (Fig. 11-37A). The histiocytes had perfectly regular, benign-appearing nuclei and an indistinct, faintly eosinophilic cytoplasm. The reticulin framework of the nodules was increased (Fig. 11-37B). In two of the patients giant cells were prominent (Fig. 11-38). A granulomatous vasculitis was present in one patient (see Fig. 11-44). In the patient taking Diabinese, the lesion disappeared when the drug was discontinued. That patient had similar lesions in a liver biopsy. The other patients were lost to follow-up. The differential diagnoses considered in these cases were large cell lymphoma, histiocytic type; Hodgkin's disease; and eosinophilic granuloma. The lack of atypism of the histiocytes and the absence of Reed-Sternberg cells ruled out lymphoma and Hodgkin's disease. The indistinct cytoplasm of the histiocytes, as well as the clinical setting, eliminated eosinophilic granuloma.

Eosinophilic Granuloma

In eosinophilic granuloma of bone the histiocytes have an abundant eosinophilic cytoplasm. They may contain varying amounts of fat and may appear as foam cells. The number of eosinophils varies (Fig. 11-39).

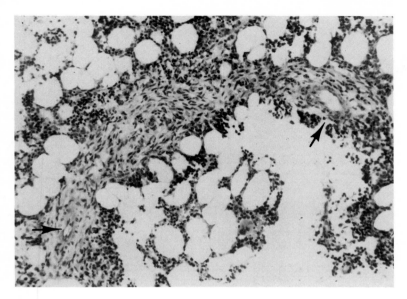

Figure 11-35
Eosinophilic fibrohistiocytic lesion, perivascular type, type II. Note the arrangement of fibrohistiocytes around blood vessels (*arrows*). (H&E, ×125.)

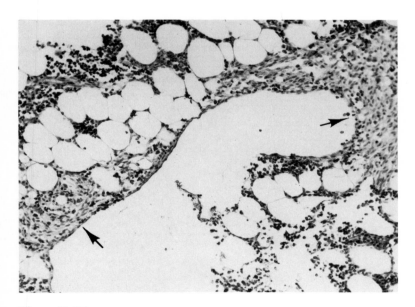

Figure 11-36
Eosinophilic fibrohistiocytic lesion, perisinusoidal type, type III. Note focal collections of fibrohistiocytes (*arrows*) adjacent to wall of sinusoid. (H&E, ×176.)

177

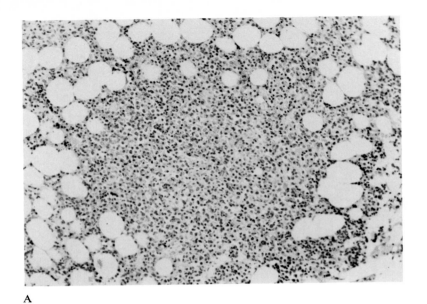

A

B

Figure 11-37
(A) Drug-related granuloma. The lesion is made up of histiocytes and lymph-ocytes. Eosinophils are also present but cannot be recognized at this power. (H&E, ×176.) (B) Same case as in A: increased reticulin framework. (Gordon-Sweets', ×192.)

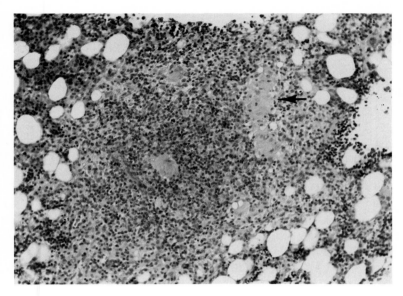

Figure 11-38
Granulomatous myelitis in patient on procainamide. Nodule made up of lymphocytes, histiocytes, and giant cells (*arrow*). Eosinophils are not visible at this magnification. (H&E, ×220.)

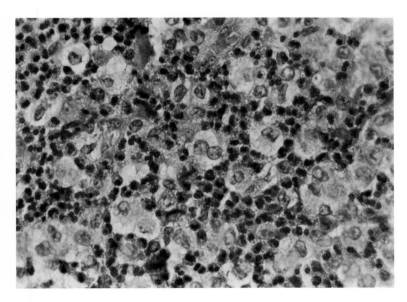

Figure 11-39
Eosinophilic granuloma. Large histiocytes with prominent, somewhat vacuolated cytoplasm; numerous interspersed eosinophils. (H&E, ×353.)

179

The precise relationship between eosinophilic granuloma, Hand-Schüller-Christian disease, and Letterer-Siwe disease is as yet unresolved. Lichtenstein [4] viewed these three diseases as related manifestations of a single histologic entity which he named *histiocytosis X*. The unitarian concept of these three diseases is supported by the presence of a distinctive, ultrastructural, rod-shaped inclusion in the cytoplasm of the proliferating histiocytes in all of them. This inclusion appears identical with the one observed in the Langerhans' cells of the epidermis [14]. Other authors consider Hand-Schüller-Christian disease to be a multifocal or systemic variant of eosinophilic granuloma unrelated to Letterer-Siwe disease [5, 8].

Vascular Lesions

Vessels are invariably seen in histologic sections of aspirated bone marrow particles. They may exhibit a variety of lesions: arteriosclerosis, thromboemboli, atheroemboli, vasculitis, and hyaline thrombi as are seen in thrombotic thrombocytopenic purpura (Figs. 11-40 to 11-45).

Miscellaneous

A variety of artifacts can be observed in histologic sections of aspirated bone marrow. Thus, fragments of skin or its components can appear in histologic sections of bone marrow particles (Fig. 11-46). It is important not to mistake sweat glands or sebaceous glands for metastatic carcinoma (Fig. 11-47). Occasionally fragments of fibrocartilage or skeletal muscle are included in the aspirate (Figs. 11-48, 11-49). When the needles, the specimen bottles, or the caps of the specimen bottles are not well cleaned, fragments from a previous marrow aspirate can be included. They can be recognized because they show elongated, darker staining nuclei associated with shrinkage of the fat cells. The iron content and histologic appearance of such a bone marrow particle may be different from that of the rest of the marrow (Fig. 11-50).

Foreign bodies of various kinds may appear in bone marrow sections. We have seen vegetable material, probably derived from a corkboard, algae, and cross sections of various parasites (Figs. 11-51 to 11-53).

Different pigments may be noted in the bone marrow. Hemosiderin is discussed in Chapter 6. Formalin pigment will be observed if the formalin is not properly buffered to neutrality. Formalin pigment exhibits double refractility and is removed by an alcoholic solution of ammonium hydroxide [7]. Malarial pigment resembles formalin pigment but is predominantly intracellular. Melanin may be seen in the marrow in metastatic melanoma. Ceroid is discussed in detail in Chapter 10. Various exogenous pigments can be observed in the bone marrow. Anthracotic pigment has been reported [1]. An example of thorotrast, a gray-brown pigment found in perivascularly located macrophages, is shown in Figure 11-54. Thorotrast emits alpha particles and can be identified by putting the slide on an x-ray film for 48 to 72 hours.

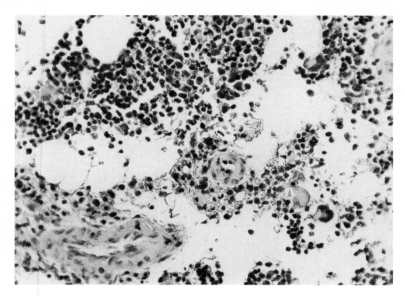

Figure 11-40
Arteriolosclerosis of bone marrow: thickened arterioles. (H&E, ×352.)

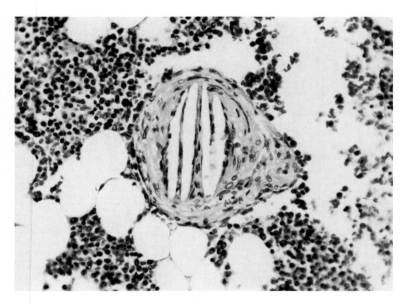

Figure 11-41
Atheromatous emboli of bone marrow. Note empty clefts from which cholesterol crystals have been dissolved by embedding process. (H&E, ×396.)

181

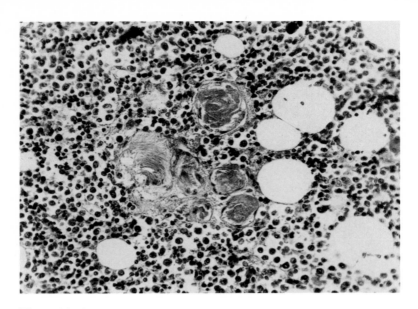

Figure 11-42
Thrombotic thrombocytopenia purpura. Hyaline thrombi in capillaries.
(H&E, ×250.)

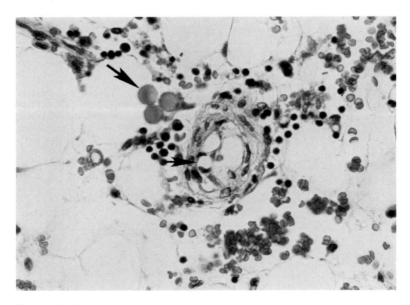

Figure 11-43
Subendothelial vacuolation (*small arrow*) after radiation therapy. The hyaline
spherules (*large arrow*) are Russell bodies. (H&E, ×635.)

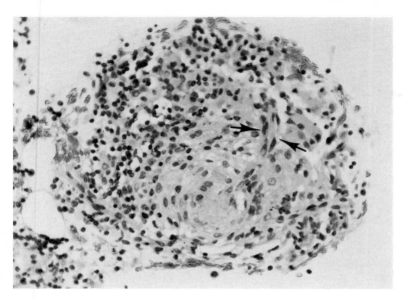

Figure 11-44
Granulomatous vasculitis in a patient with drug-related granulomatous inflammation of bone marrow (*vessel between arrows*). (H&E, ×366.)

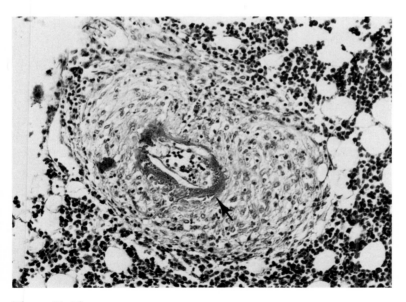

Figure 11-45
Periarteritis nodosa of bone marrow. Fibrinoid necrosis of vessel wall (*arrow*) and perivascular histiocytic infiltration. (H&E, ×198.)

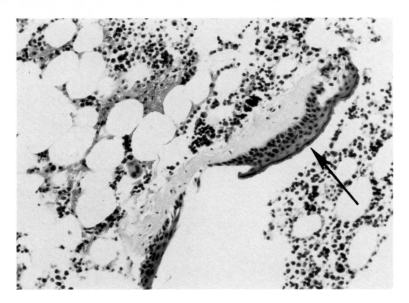

Figure 11-46
Fragment of skin (*arrow*) included in bone marrow preparation. (H&E, ×195.)

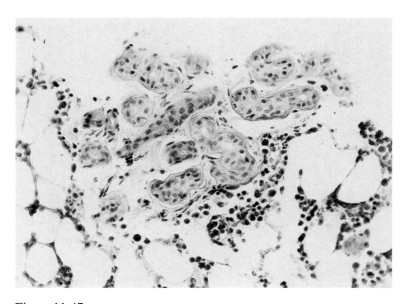

Figure 11-47
Sweat glands artifactually included in bone marrow preparation. They should not be mistaken for metastatic carcinoma. (H&E, ×352.)

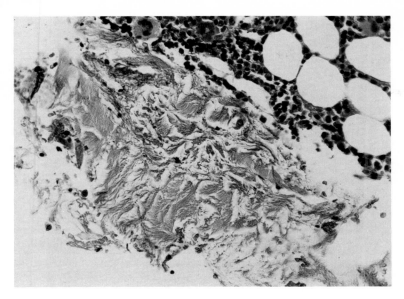

Figure 11-48
Appearance of fibrocartilage in bone marrow aspirate. (H&E, ×374.)

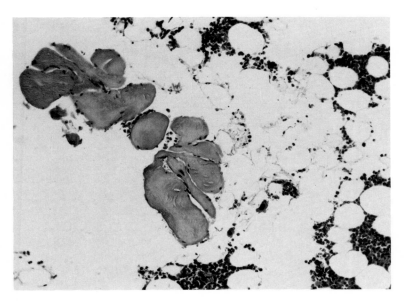

Figure 11-49
Appearance of skeletal muscle in bone marrow aspirate. (H&E, ×220.)

185

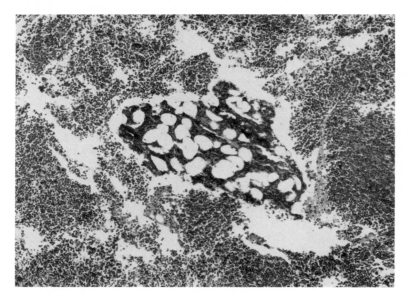

Figure 11-50
Appearance of dried-out bone marrow particle from previous aspiration (improperly cleaned needle or specimen jar). Present bone marrow is markedly hypercellular whereas dried-out particle is normocellular. (H&E, ×78.)

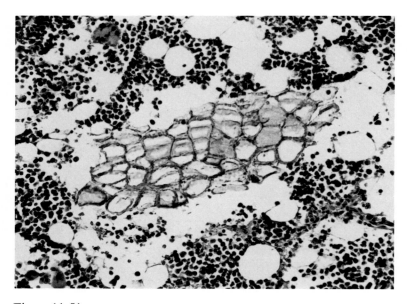

Figure 11-51
Artifact: vegetable cells (rectangular appearance of cell walls) probably derived from corkboard. (H&E, ×214.)

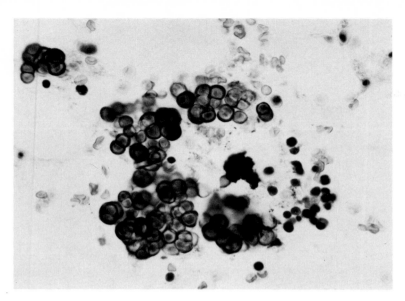

Figure 11-52
Artifact: brown septate bodies, probably algae from contaminated water or stain. (H&E, ×635.)

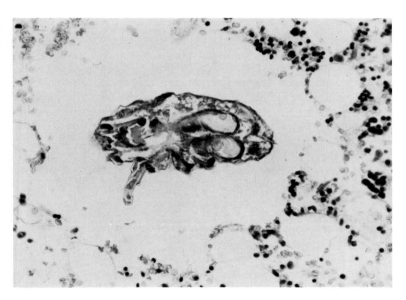

Figure 11-53
Cross section of insect artifactually included in bone marrow preparation. (H&E, ×396.)

187

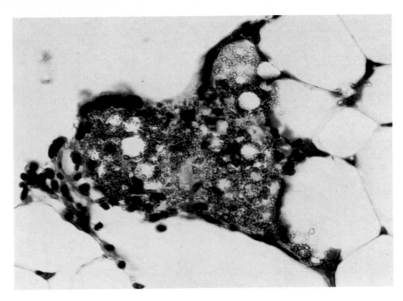

Figure 11-54
Thorotrast granules in bone marrow macrophages. (H&E, ×530.)

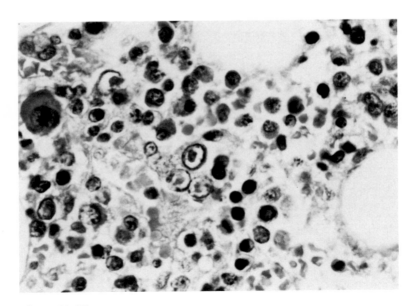

Figure 11-55
Eosinophilic intranuclear inclusions surrounded by clear halo. (H&E, ×634.)

We have seen striking eosinophilic intranuclear inclusions in bone marrow sections kindly sent to us by Dr. Lucy Rorke of the Philadelphia General Hospital. This bone marrow aspirate was obtained from a 72-year-old black man with a history of alcoholic cirrhosis and pulmonary tuberculosis. On admission, the patient was febrile and severely anemic. He improved markedly with transfusions and isoniazid. The inclusions were eosinophilic, round to oval, and situated within enlarged vesicular nuclei with an accentuated nuclear membrane (Fig. 11-55). No cytoplasmic inclusions were seen. The nature of the cells containing the inclusions could not be determined. The inclusions resembled those seen in herpesvirus infections. However, it is important to remember that in addition to viral infections, intranuclear inclusions can be found in heavy metal poisoning. The significance of the inclusions in this patient has not been determined.

References

1. Askanazy, M. Knockenmark. In F. Henke and O. Lubarsch (Eds.), *Handbuch der speziellen pathologischen Anatomie und Histologie.* Berlin: Springer, 1927. Vol. I, pt. 2, p. 853.
2. Hudson, P., Jr., and Robertson, G. M., Jr. Demonstration of mineral oil in splenic "lipid granulomas" (abstract). *Lab. Invest.* 15:1134, 1966.
3. Lewis, S. M., and Szur, L. Malignant myelosclerosis. *Br. Med. J.* 2:472, 1963.
4. Lichtenstein, L. Histiocytosis X: Integration of eosinophilic granuloma of bone, Letterer-Siwe disease and Schüller-Christian disease as related to manifestations of a single nosologic entity. *Arch. Pathol.* 56:84, 1953.
5. Lieberman, P. H., Jones, C. R., Dargeon, H. W. K., and Begg, C. F. A reappraisal of eosinophilic granuloma of bone, Hand-Schüller-Christian syndrome and Letterer-Siwe syndrome. *Medicine* (Baltimore) 48:375, 1969.
6. Lubin, J., Rozen, S., and Rywlin, A. M. Malignant myelosclerosis. *Arch. Intern. Med.* 136:141, 1976.
7. Luna, L. G. *Manual of Histologic Staining Methods of the Armed Forces Institute of Pathology* (3rd ed.). New York: McGraw-Hill, 1968. P. 179.
8. Nyholm, K. Eosinophilic xanthomatous granulomatosis and Letterer-Siwe's disease. *Acta Pathol. Microbiol. Scand.* [A] Suppl. 216, 1971.
9. Patakfalvi, B., Csete, B., and Horvath, T. Familial myelofibrosis. *Haematologica* 3:217, 1969.
10. Rohr, K. *Das menschliche Knochenmark* (3rd ed.). Stuttgart: Thieme, 1960. Pp. 359, 488.
11. Rywlin, A. M., Hoffman, E. P., and Ortega, R. S. Eosinophilic fibrohistiocytic lesion of bone marrow: A distinctive new morphologic finding, probably related to drug hypersensitivity. *Blood* 40:464, 1972.
12. Rywlin, A. M., Lopez-Gomez, A., Tachmes, P., and Pardo, V. Ceroid histiocytosis of spleen in hyperlipemia: Relationship to the syndrome of the sea-blue histiocyte. *Am. J. Clin. Pathol.* 56:572, 1971.

13. Rywlin, A. M., and Ortega, R. S. Lipid granulomas of the bone marrow. *Am. J. Clin. Pathol.* 57:457, 1972.
14. Tarnowski, W. M., and Hashimoto, K. Langerhans' cell granules in histiocytosis X: The epidermal Langerhans' cell as a macrophage. *Arch. Dermatol.* 96:298, 1967.

12 Some Aspects of Bone Pathology

The examination of needle or surgical biopsies of bone marrow gives the hematopathologist an opportunity to examine osseous tissue. It therefore is appropriate to review briefly some aspects of bone pathology likely to be encountered in such biopsies. Additional information can be obtained in more detailed monographs [1, 3, 6].

A biopsy usually shows cortical bone with tendinous insertions and spongy (cancellous) bone, composed of trabeculae traversing the marrow. The bone trabeculae are made up of mature (lamellar) bone. An orderly, parallel arrangement of the lamellae is characteristic of mature bone, and its appearance can be accentuated by decreasing the aperture of the iris diaphragm or by viewing the trabeculae through crossed Nicol prisms (Fig. 12-1). In contrast to mature bone, in immature bone (metaplastic bone, coarsely woven bone, fiber bone), the collagen lamellae run in all directions and the osteocytes are larger and more numerous (see Figs. 7-12, 11-1, 12-7). The surface of the bone trabeculae is covered by endosteum that normally consists of a single layer of scanty, inconspicuous, flattened, endotheliumlike cells (Fig. 12-2). Adjacent to the bone trabeculae is the hematopoietic marrow. Occasionally the hematopoietic marrow is separated from the endosteal surface of the bone trabeculae by fatty marrow (Fig. 12-3).

Osteosclerosis

Osteosclerosis refers to the formation of more bone than is normally present per unit volume of tissue. The newly formed bone may be immature in type (see p. 154). Immature bone may form endosteally by apposition to preexisting bone trabeculae, or it may arise through metaplasia in foci of myelofibrosis (see Fig. 11-1). As the immature bone ages, it is remodeled and takes on the appearance of mature, i.e., lamellar bone. Osteosclerosis is usually secondary to myelofibrosis (see p. 154). However, in the congenital osteoscleroses, such as osteopetrosis, myelofibrosis does not precede the osteosclerosis, which is due to a primary defect in bone resorption.

Osteoporosis

In osteoporosis there is a decrease in the amount of bone per unit volume of tissue (Fig. 12-4B). Radiologically the bone is less dense than normal. The individual bone trabeculae are thinner and more widely separated (Fig. 12-5); otherwise they are histologically unremarkable. The endosteal surface of the trabeculae appears normal, and it is impossible

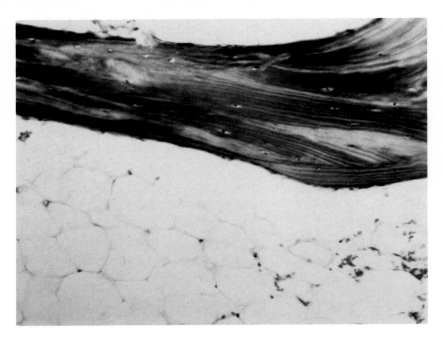

Figure 12-1
Bone trabecula made up of mature (lamellar) bone. Note characteristic
parallel arrangement of lamellae, accentuated by Nicol prisms. (H&E,
×130.)

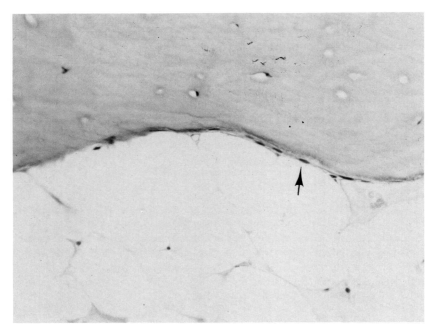

Figure 12-2
Flattened, endotheliumlike endosteal cells lining bone trabecula (*arrow*).
(H&E, ×260.)

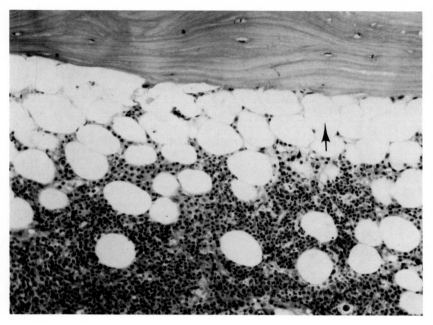

Figure 12-3
Fatty marrow (*arrow*) between bone trabecula and hematopoietic marrow.
(H&E, ×130.)

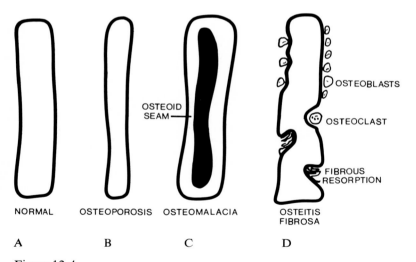

Figure 12-4
Appearance of bone trabeculae in various forms of bone atrophy. (A) Normal bone trabecula. (B) Osteoporosis: Bone trabecula is thinner than normal; endosteal surface is smooth. (C) Osteomalacia: Note osteoid seam and calcified center. (D) Osteitis fibrosa: Note fibrous resorption of bone, accompanied by increased osteoclastic and osteoblastic activity.

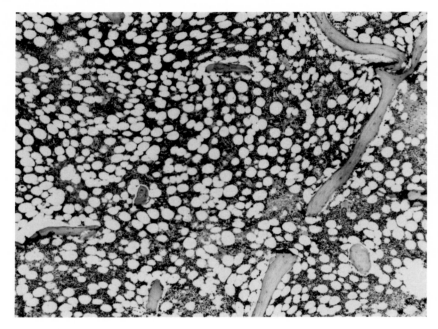

Figure 12-5
Osteoporosis. Thin and widely separated bone trabeculae. (H&E, ×40.)

to demonstrate a decreased number of osteoblasts by usual technics. Osteoid seams are inconspicuous and osteoclastic activity is not increased. The bone marrow is normal. Increased numbers of mast cells have been reported [2]. These changes in trabecular bone are accompanied by resorption and cancellous transformation of the compact cortical bone.

Osteoporosis can be generalized or localized. Generalized osteoporosis may be primary, or it may occur secondary to Cushing's syndrome, hyperthyroidism, and the prolonged administration of corticosteroids or heparin. Localized osteoporosis is a form of disuse atrophy.

Osteomalacia

The histopathologic landmark of osteomalacia is the osteoid seam (Figs. 12-4C, 12-6), which appears in bone trabeculae as a rim of noncalcified protein matrix surrounding a central calcified core. The osteoid seam is seen in decalcified, hematoxylin and eosin-stained sections because it appears pinker and paler than the centrally located calcified bone. Osteoid seams are recognized much more easily in undecalcified tissue sections stained with alizarin red or with von Kossa's silver stain (see Fig.

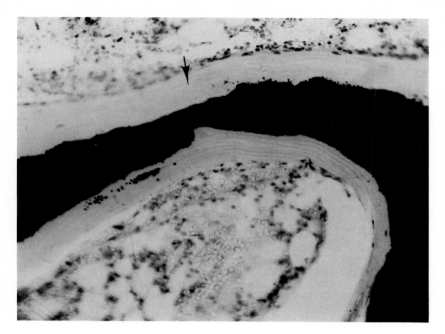

Figure 12-6
Osteomalacia. Bone trabecula exhibits central, calcified black area (precipitated metallic silver) and uncalcified osteoid seam (*arrow*). (von Kossa,
×130.)

12-6). The sodium alizarinsulfonate forms a dye lake with calcium car-
bonate and phosphate [5]. In the von Kossa reaction the calcium in
tissues is replaced by silver from a solution of silver nitrate. The silver is
reduced to metallic silver through exposure to light and appears as a
black deposit in tissue, replacing the calcium [5].

The osteoid seams are associated with prominent osteoblastic activity.
Osteoclasts are not increased in osteomalacia. While fully developed
osteomalacia is easily recognized, early cases require morphometric
studies. Narrow osteoid seams not exceeding 3μ in width may be seen in
occasional trabeculae in normal bone. For the evaluation of minor degrees of osteomalacia, it is important to determine not only the width of
the osteoid seams but also the extent to which trabeculae are surrounded
by them.

In osteomalacia, normal resorption of bone is countered by the laying
down of osteoid that does not calcify because of a lack of vitamin D or
calcium. Vitamin D and calcium deficiencies may result from an inadequate dietary intake or from intestinal malabsorption. Enlarged osteoid
seams may also develop in phosphate deficiency, hypophosphatasia, and
renal osteodystrophy.

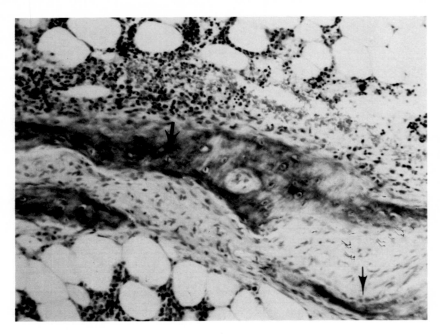

Figure 12-7
Osteitis fibrosa. Note fibrosis, formation of immature (metaplastic) bone
(*thick arrow*), and row of osteoblasts (*thin arrow*). (H&E, ×130.)

Osteitis Fibrosa

The term *osteitis fibrosa* is used to describe the histologic findings in
hyperparathyroidism. These consist of endosteal fibrosis that results in
tonguelike projections of fibrous tissue which penetrate into bone trabeculae and cause resorption (Figs. 12-4D, 12-7; see also Fig. 1-7). As the
disease progresses the endosteal fibrosis extends throughout the marrow,
replacing hematopoietic and fatty marrow. Associated with the endosteal
fibrosis is a proliferation of osteoclasts that resorb the trabecular bone,
creating Howship's lacunae. Occasionally, in advanced cases, the proliferation of fibrous tissue with many osteoclasts creates a tumorlike mass
that is identical histologically with giant cell tumors of bone. In addition
to fibrous and osteoclastic resorption of bone, a bone biopsy may reveal
attempts at bone regeneration resulting in the formation of immature
bone (see Fig. 12-7). Active osteoblastic proliferation with formation
of osteoid seams may also be observed; the latter are not as wide as in
osteomalacia.

Needle biopsy of bone and marrow, because of its simplicity, should
be performed in cases of hypercalcemia. Metastatic carcinoma, multiple
myeloma, sarcoidosis, and hyperparathyroidism are among the causes

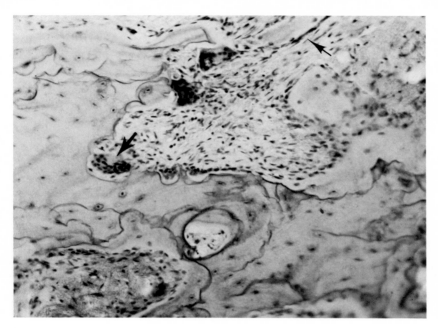

Figure 12-8
Paget's disease. Note fibrosis of marrow, osteoclastic (*thick arrow*) and osteoblastic (*thin arrow*) activity, and mosaic appearance of bone trabeculae
due to cementing lines. (H&E, ×260.)

of hypercalcemia and may all be diagnosed by bone biopsy. It has been
stated that the majority of patients with hyperparathyroidism have no
demonstrable bone disease [1]. This is true when bone is examined by
roentgenograms alone. When bone biopsy and alkaline phosphatase
determination are added as parameters for recognizing bone disease,
however, the number of cases of hyperparathyroidism with demonstrable
bone disease increases. How often one can expect diagnostic findings
from needle biopsies of bone in cases of proved hyperparathyroidism is
unknown at the present time.

The bone changes found in chronic renal disease exhibit a mixed oste-
opathy, i.e., they consist in varying proportions of osteitis fibrosa, osteomalacia, and osteosclerosis. When the pathologist sees osteitis fibrosa
associated with significantly wide osteoid seams, suggesting the presence
of osteomalacia, he should suspect renal osteodystrophy.

Paget's Disease

Paget's disease is characterized histologically by: (1) increased vascularity and fibrosis of the bone marrow; (2) increased osteoclastic activ-

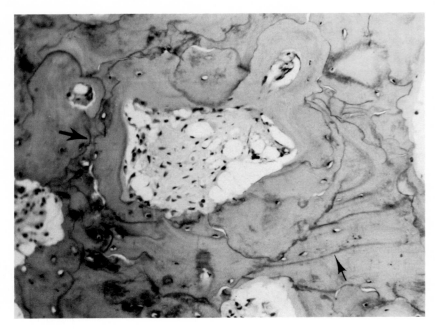

Figure 12-9
Paget's disease of bone. Note two types of cementing lines: (1) thin and wavy lines of erosion (*thick arrow*) and (2) thicker and straighter resting lines (*thin arrow*). Osteoclastic and osteoblastic activity is not prominent. Fibrous marrow begins to be replaced by fatty marrow. Paget's disease is less active than that shown in Figure 12-8. (H&E, ×130.)

ity, resulting in a scalloped appearance of the trabecular surfaces; (3) osteoblastic activity with formation of metaplastic and, later, lamellar bone; and (4) widened trabeculae exhibiting a mosaic appearance.

Increased vascularity, edema, and fibrosis of the marrow occur first. They are closely followed by a rise in osteoclastic and osteoblastic activity (Fig. 12-8). As the disease progresses, the trabeculae exhibit a typical mosaic appearance caused by the presence of numerous cementing lines criss-crossing the trabeculae (Figs. 12-8, 12-9). Cementing lines are more basophilic than the rest of the bone. The cause of this basophilia is not well understood [4]. There are two types of cementing lines: resting lines and lines of erosion (reversal lines). The resting lines are thicker and straighter than the lines of erosion, which are thin and wavy. Cementing lines are thought to represent clues to past events in bone trabeculae. Resting lines are evidence of past osteoblastic activity and are formed during a local pause between two periods of bone formation. Lines of erosion result from the confluence of Howship's lacunae and thus represent evidence of past osteoclastic activity. They are formed during a pause between bone resorption and bone formation. In the burnt-out or final phase of Paget's disease, the fibrous marrow is replaced by fatty or hematopoietic marrow, while the trabeculae retain their mosaic appearance.

The mosaic pattern of the trabeculae is highly specific for Paget's disease. Minor degrees of mosaicism may be seen in fibrous dysplasia and osteitis fibrosa. As in all bone diseases, the final diagnosis must rest on a combination of clinical, chemical, radiologic, and histologic data.

References

1. Collins, D. H. *Pathology of Bone*. London: Butterworth, 1966.
2. Frame, B., and Nixon, R. K. Bone-marrow mast cells in osteoporosis of aging. *N. Engl. J. Med.* 279:626, 1968.
3. Jaffe, H. L. *Metabolic, Degenerative, and Inflammatory Diseases of Bones and Joints*. Philadelphia: Lea & Febiger, 1972.
4. Rutishauer, E., and Majno, G. Physiopathology of bone tissue: The osteocytes and fundamental substance. *Bull. Hosp. Joint Dis.* 12:468, 1951.
5. Thompson, S. W. *Selected Histochemical and Histopathological Methods*. Springfield, Ill.: Thomas, 1966.
6. Weinmann, J. P., and Sicher, H. *Bone and Bones. Fundamentals of Bone Biology* (2nd ed.). St. Louis: Mosby, 1955.

Appendix
Staining Procedures

1. Giemsa Stain for Tissue Sections (Wolbach's Modification)

Fixation

Zenker fixative is best; 10% neutral buffered formalin may be used. Stains decalcified tissue poorly (see note).

Objective

1. To recognize blast cells, characterized by a narrow deep blue rim of cytoplasm, round to oval nuclei with prominent nucleoli, and large nuclear-cytoplasmic ratios.
2. To stain mast cell granules.
3. To accentuate plasma cells and eosinophils.

Reagents

GIEMSA STOCK SOLUTION
Giemsa powder	1.0 gm
Methyl alcohol	66.0 ml
Glycerin	66.0 ml

Add glycerin to Giemsa powder. Put in 60°C oven for 2 hours. Add methyl alcohol.

ROSIN STOCK SOLUTION
White rosin	10.0 gm
Absolute alcohol	100.00 ml

GIEMSA WORKING SOLUTION
Giemsa stock solution	1.25 ml
Absolute methyl alcohol	1.25 ml
Distilled water	50.00 ml

ROSIN WORKING SOLUTION
Rosin stock solution	5.0 ml
95% alcohol	40.0 ml

Source

Giemsa powder: National Biologic Stains and Reagents Department, Allied Chemical Corp., P.O. Box 431, Morristown, N.J. 07960

Procedure

1. Deparaffinize and hydrate to distilled water.
2. Remove mercury precipitates with iodine and 5% sodium thiosulfate if Zenker fixed.

3. Rinse well in distilled water.
4. Place in working solution of Giemsa stain overnight.
5. Differentiate in rosin alcohol until sections assume a purplish pink color. Check under microscope for cytoplasmic and nuclear detail.
6. Absolute ethyl alcohol—3 changes.
7. Clear with xylol.
8. Mount with Permount or balsam.

Results

Nuclei	blue
Collagen and other tissue elements	pink to rose

NOTE: Giemsa stain takes much better if tissue has acid pH.
Better results are obtained with decalcified sections if Cal-Ex (SO-C-190, Fisher Scientific Co., 711 Forbes Ave., Pittsburgh, Pa. 15219) is used for decalcification and the staining solution containing the slides is heated to 60°C for 30 minutes before differentiation.

Reference

1. Luna, L. G. *Manual of Histologic Staining Methods of the Armed Forces Institute of Pathology* (3rd ed.). New York: McGraw-Hill, 1968. Pp. 119–120.

2. Gomori's Iron Reaction

Fixation

Cell block of bone marrow particles formalin fixed, Paraplast embedded.

Objective

To demonstrate hemosiderin granules.

Reagents

20% HYDROCHLORIC ACID STOCK SOLUTION
Hydrochloric acid, concentrated	20.0 ml
Distilled water	80.0 ml

10% POTASSIUM FERROCYANIDE STOCK SOLUTION
Potassium ferrocyanide	10.0 ml
Distilled water	100.0 ml

HYDROCHLORIC ACID–POTASSIUM FERROCYANIDE WORKING SOLUTION
Hydrochloric acid stock solution	50.0 ml
Potassium ferrocyanide stock solution	50.0 ml

Mix just before use.

NUCLEAR-FAST RED (KERNECHTROT) WORKING SOLUTION
Nuclear-fast red	0.1 gm
Aluminum sulfate solution 5% aqueous	100.0 ml

Dissolve nuclear-fast red in solution of aluminum sulfate with the aid of heat; cool and filter. Add as a preservative a crystal of thymol. Keeps well at room temperature. Can be reused.

Source

Potassium ferrocyanide: J. T. Baker Chemical Co., Phillipsburg, N.J. 08865.

Nuclear-fast red (Kernechtrot): Roboz Surgical Instrument Co., 810 18th St., N.W., Washington, D.C. 20006.

Procedure

1. Hydrate sections through xylol and alcohols to distilled water.
2. Place slides in hydrochloric acid–potassium ferrocyanide solution for 30 minutes.
3. Rinse thoroughly in distilled water.
4. Counterstain in nuclear-fast red solution for 5 minutes.
5. Rinse in distilled water.
6. Dehydrate in 95% alcohol and absolute alcohol, clear in xylol.
7. Mount with Permount or balsam.

Results

Hemosiderin	bright blue
Nuclei	red
Cytoplasm	light pink

Reference

1. Gomori, G. Microtechnical demonstration of iron. *Am. J. Pathol.* 12: 655, 1936.

3. Gordon-Sweets' Method for Reticulin Fibers

Fixation

Tissue may be fixed with any of the usual fixatives. Paraplast-embedded or frozen sections may be used.

Objective

To demonstrate reticulin fibers.

Reagents

SILVER SOLUTION

To 5 ml of 10% aqueous silver nitrate add 28% ammonia water drop by drop until the precipitate formed is just dissolved (approximately 0.4 ml). Then add 5 ml of 3% sodium hydroxide, followed by 28% ammonia water until the solution is clear. Make up to 50 ml with distilled water.

ACIDIFIED POTASSIUM PERMANGANATE

0.5% potassium permanganate	95.0 ml
3.0% sulfuric acid	5.0 ml

REDUCING SOLUTION

37% formaldehyde	10.0 ml
Distilled water	90.0 ml

GOLD CHLORIDE SOLUTION

1% gold chloride solution	10.0 ml
Distilled water	40.0 ml

SODIUM THIOSULFATE SOLUTION

Sodium thiosulfate	5.0 gm
Distilled water	100.0 ml

FERRIC AMMONIUM SULFATE (MORDANT)

Ferric ammonium sulfate	2.0 gm
Distilled water	100.0 ml

NUCLEAR-FAST RED (KERNECHTROT) SOLUTION

Nuclear-fast red	0.1 gm
5% aluminum sulfate solution	100.0 ml

Source

Any source.

Procedure

1. Hydrate sections through xylol and alcohols to distilled water.
2. Oxidize for 1 to 3 minutes in acidified potassium permanganate.
3. Rinse with distilled water.
4. Bleach in 1% oxalic acid for 1 minute.
5. Rinse well with distilled water at least 3 times.
6. Apply mordant solution for 2 to 10 minutes. Rinse well in water.

7. Impregnate with silver solution 5 to 30 seconds, until sections appear transparent.
8. Rinse well in several changes of distilled water.
9. Reduce in 10% aqueous formalin.
10. Wash in tap water for 3 changes.
11. Tone with gold chloride solution for 2 minutes.
12. Wash in tap water for 3 changes.
13. Fix in 5% sodium thiosulfate for 3 minutes.
14. Wash well in tap water for 2 minutes.
15. Counterstain with nuclear-fast red solution for 5 minutes.
16. Wash briefly with tap water.
17. Dehydrate in 95% alcohol and absolute alcohol, clear in xylol.
18. Mount with Permount or balsam.

Results

Reticulin fibers	black to deep purple
Nerve fibers	black
Elastic fibers	black
Collagen	yellowish brown

References

1. Culling, C. F. A. *Handbook of Histopathological Techniques* (2nd ed.). London: Butterworth, 1963. Pp. 347–348.
2. Lynch, M. J., Raphael, S. S., Mellor, L. D., Spare, P. D., and Inwood, M. J. H. *Medical Laboratory Technology and Clinical Pathology* (2nd ed.). Philadelphia: Saunders, 1969. P. 113.

4. Methyl Green–Pyronine Stain

Fixation

Cell block of formalin-fixed, Paraplast-embedded bone marrow particles. Smears fixed in 10% formalin methanol for 10 minutes.

Objective

To bring out RNA, which is pyroninophilic and stains red. This stain brings out blast cells and plasma cells by staining their cytoplasm red. The red cytoplasmic rim of blasts is equivalent to the blue rims seen with the Giemsa stain. It is a good nucleolar stain.

Reagents

METHYL GREEN–PYRONINE

Pyronine	0.25 gm
Methyl green	0.75 gm
Phosphate buffer, pH 5.3	100.00 ml
To this add:	
0.5% phenol solution	0.5 ml
1.0% resorcinol	2.5 ml

Methyl green–pyronine stain is relatively stable. It requires 2 to 3 days to ripen and will last 3 to 6 months at room temperature. Can be reused if refrigerated when not in use.

PHOSPHATE BUFFER MIXTURE

0.2 M disodium phosphate (Na_2HPO_4)	52.5 ml
0.1 M citric acid	47.5 ml

(Both of the above made up in 25% methyl alcohol.) If these proportions do not give a pH of 5.3, the solution must be adjusted to pH 5.3.

Source

Methyl green GA: Chroma-Gesellschaft, distributed by Roboz Surgical Instrument Co., 810 18th St., N.W., Washington, D.C. 20006

Pyronin GS: Chroma-Gesellschaft, distributed by Roboz Surgical Instrument Co., Washington, D.C.

Resorcinol: Fisher Scientific Co., 711 Forbes Ave., Pittsburgh, Pa. 15219

Procedure

1. Hydrate sections through xylol and alcohols to distilled water.
2. Stain in methyl green–pyronine reagent ½ to 2 minutes. As the solutions age, extend the time.
3. Differentiate in 2 changes of distilled water.
4. Dehydrate rapidly in 2 changes of acetone. If acetone removes too much of the red stain, blot dry with bibulous paper.
5. Clear in xylol.
6. Mount with Permount or balsam.

Results

Cytoplasmic and nucleolar ribonucleic acid	red
Plasma cell cytoplasm	red
Cytoplasm of blasts	red

References

1. Culling, C. F. A. *Handbook of Histopathological Techniques* (2nd ed.). London: Butterworth, 1963. Pp. 219–220.
2. McManus, J. F. A., and Mowry, R. W. *Staining Methods Histologic and Histochemical.* New York: Hoeber Div., Harper & Row, 1960. P. 76.

5. Naphthol AS-D Chloroacetate (Leder) Stain

Fixation

Formalin-fixed and Paraplast-embedded bone marrow particles.

Objective

To demonstrate neutrophilic and mast cell granules.

Reagents: Stock Solutions

4% PARAROSANILINE HYDROCHLORIDE

Pararosaniline hydrochloride	1.0 gm
Distilled water	20.0 ml
Hydrochloric acid, concentrated	5.0 ml

Gently warm solution after mixing, filter, and refrigerate.

4% SODIUM NITRITE SOLUTION

Sodium nitrite	2.0 gm
Distilled water	50.0 ml

MICHAELIS VERONAL ACETATE BUFFER STOCK SOLUTION

Sodium acetate	4.857 gm
Sodium diethylbarbiturate	7.357 gm
Distilled water	250.0 ml

MICHAELIS VERONAL ACETATE WORKING SOLUTION (pH 7.42)

Veronal acetate buffer stock solution	42.4 ml
0.1 N hydrochloric acid	37.6 ml

ESTERASE SUBSTRATE SOLUTION

(Prepare just before use.)

Naphthol AS-D chloroacetate	20.0 mg
N,N dimethylformamide	2.0 ml

STAINING SOLUTION

4% pararosaniline	0.1 ml
4% sodium nitrite	0.1 ml

Mix well. Wait 60 seconds until straw color develops. Add 60.0 ml veronal acetate working buffer solution with pH 7.42. Adjust pH to 6.3 with 1.0 N HCl, about 5 drops. Add 2.0 ml esterase substrate solution. Mix, then filter. Solution should be milky pink before filtration, light pink after. Staining solution is now ready to use.

Source

Naphthol AS-D chloroacetate: Sigma Chemical Co., P.O. Box 14508, St. Louis, Mo. 63178

Pararosaniline: Sigma Chemical Co., St. Louis, Mo.
N-N dimethylformamide: Sigma Chemical Co., St. Louis, Mo.

Procedure

1. Deparaffinize and hydrate to distilled water.
2. Incubate at room temperature 30 minutes in staining solutions.
3. Rinse well with distilled water, 3 changes.
4. Counterstain with Mayer's hematoxylin for 5 minutes.
5. Rinse under running tap water for 20 minutes.
6. Dehydrate and clear with xylol.
7. Mount with Permount or balsam.

Results

Neutrophilic granules	scarlet
Mast cell granules	scarlet
Nuclei	blue

Reference

1. Leder, L. D.   Uber die selektive fermentcytochemische Darstellung von neutrophilen myeloischen Zellen und Gewebsmastzellen im Paraffinschnitt. *Klin. Wochenschr.* 42:533, 1964.

6. Wright-Giemsa Stain for Smears

Fixation
Smears of blood or bone marrow air dried or fixed in methyl alcohol.

Objective
Differentiation of hematologic elements.

Reagents

WRIGHT STOCK STAIN
Wright stain powder	0.3 gm
Glycerol (neutral)	3.0 ml
Methyl alcohol, absolute	97.0 ml

Grind the powder with mortar and pestle. Add glycerol and again thoroughly grind. Add methyl alcohol and mix. Allow to stand overnight in a tightly stoppered flask. Filter and use after 2 days. Age improves the stain.

GIEMSA STOCK STAIN
Giemsa powder	1.0 gm
Methyl alcohol	66.0 ml
Glycerin	66.0 ml

Add glycerin to Giemsa powder. Place in 60°C oven for ½ to 2 hours. Mix with methyl alcohol. Do not filter until after diluted for use. Stock solution improves with age.

GIEMSA WORKING STAIN
Stock Giemsa stain	2.0 ml
Distilled water, pH 6.5	50.0 ml

Source
Wright stain powder: Harleco Corp., 60th & Woodland Ave., Philadelphia, Pa. 19143

Giemsa powder: National Biologic Stains and Reagents Department, Allied Chemical Corp., P.O. Box 431, Morristown, N.J. 07960

Giemsa stock solution may be ordered already prepared from Harleco Corp., 60th & Woodland Ave., Philadelphia, Pa. 19143

Procedure
1. Cover the dried or methyl alcohol–fixed film completely with Wright stock stain for 1 to 2 minutes.
2. Add distilled water (pH 6.5) to the stain, drop by drop, until a greenish, metallic sheen or scum appears on the surface. Stain 2 to 5 minutes. The neutrophilic granules should stain lilac, the eosinophilic granules bright red, and the basophilic granules deep blue.

3. Place slides in distilled water horizontally and slowly enough to allow the metallic scum to float off. Wash briefly but briskly with fresh water to remove excess stain (approximately 5 to 10 seconds).
4. Place slides in Coplin jar with Giemsa working solution for 5 minutes. Check under the microscope for cytoplasmic and nuclear detail.
5. Rinse off excess stain with distilled water (3 changes).
6. Clean back of slides, air dry or blot dry, and clear with xylol.
7. Mount with Permount or balsam.

Results

Chromatin	red or purple red
Cytoplasm	blue
Erythrocytes	light pink
Nuclei	deep purple to violet
Granules in neutrophils	lilac
Eosinophils	bright red
Basophils	deep blue

The color of erythrocytes varies with the pH of the diluting water, from pink at pH 6.0 through yellowish pink at 6.5, pinkish or grayish yellow at 6.8, grayish yellow to greenish yellow or even gray blue at 7.0 to 7.2. Differentiation with distilled water, which is often faintly acid, or with very dilute (0.05–0.1%) acetic acid displaces the color of erythrocytes from the gray blue toward the pink limit of the color series above.

References

1. Lillie, R. D. *Histopathologic Technic and Practical Histochemistry* (3rd ed.). New York: Blakiston Div., McGraw-Hill, 1965. Pp. 340, 467.
2. War Department Technical Manual, October, 1946. Pp. 41–42.

7. Periodic Acid–Schiff (PAS) Reaction

Fixation

Absolute ethyl alcohol fixative (10% buffered formalin may be used).

Objective

To demonstrate glycogen and substances containing polysaccharides. After treatment of the tissue with diastase, PAS positivity of glycogen disappears. Glycogen is water soluble, and absolute alcohol is the preferred fixative.

Reagents

ALCOHOLIC PERIODIC ACID (OXIDATION AGENT)

Periodic acid	4.0 gm
Distilled water	100.0 ml
0.2 M sodium acetate buffer	50.0 ml
100% ethyl alcohol	350.0 ml

ACID-REDUCING RINSE

Potassium iodide	2.0 gm
Sodium thiosulfate	2.0 gm
Distilled water	40.0 ml
100% ethyl alcohol	60.0 ml
0.1 N hydrochloric acid	2.0 ml

SCHIFF'S REAGENT

Basic fuchsin	2.0 gm
Boiling distilled water	400.0 ml
(cool to 50°C and filter)	
2 N hydrochloric acid	10.0 ml
Potassium metabisulfite	4.0 gm

Stopper and let cool in dark overnight. Next morning filter and add 1 gm or more of Norite "A" and shake for 1 minute. Filter through 2 filter papers. Add up to 5 ml of 2 N HCl until stain drying on slide does not turn pink. Store in dark bottle in refrigerator.

SULFUROUS ACID RINSE

10% potassium metabisulfite	80.0 ml
Hydrochloric acid	20.0 ml
Distilled water	2000.0 ml

2 N HYDROCHLORIC ACID

Hydrochloric acid	167.0 ml
Distilled water	833.0 ml

Use only glass container and glass instruments.

Source

Any source.

Procedure

1. Deparaffinize and carry sections to 70% alcohol.
2. Place sections in alcoholic periodic acid solution for 5 minutes.
3. Rinse sections in 2 changes of 70% alcohol.
4. Place sections in reducing rinse for 1 minute.
5. Rinse sections in 2 changes of 70% alcohol.
6. Place in Schiff's reagent for 15 minutes or more.
7. Place sections in 3 changes of sulfurous acid rinse, 5 minutes each.
8. Wash well in water.
9. Counterstain with Harris' hematoxylin for 3 minutes.
10. Rinse in tap water.
11. Differentiate in 1% acid alcohol.
12. Wash in tap water.
13. Blue in 1% ammonia water.
14. Wash in running water for 5 minutes.
15. Dehydrate, clear, and mount.

Results

Materials staining red to purple are said to be PAS positive. Stains mast cells and intracytoplasmic, intranuclear, and interstitial IgM and IgA deposits.

Carbohydrates (glycogen, polysaccharides), intestinal epithelial mucus, capsules, and the walls of fungi	magenta to purple
Basement membranes (kidney and skin)	reddish purple

Reference

1. Culling, C. F. A. *Handbook of Histopathological Techniques* (2nd ed.). London: Butterworth, 1963. Pp. 228–246.

Index

Myeloslerosis, 153
  chronic, lymphoid type, 125
  malignant, 155, 156
Myelosis
  erythremic, 50–51
    differential diagnosis of, 51, 52
    dyserythropoiesis in, 50
    hemosiderin in, 57
  megakaryocytic
    acute, 36
    hypercellular marrow in, 25
    megakaryocytes in, 36, 38
Myositis, granulocytic hyperplasia
    in, 64

Naphthol AS-D chloroacetate stain,
    208–209
Necrosis of tissue, granulocytic
    hyperplasia in, 64
Necrotic fat cells, 155, 158
  differential diagnosis of, 169
Needle aspiration. *See* Aspiration
    of marrow
Needle biopsy, 8–10
Neoplasms
  granulocytic hyperplasia in, 64
  megakaryocytes in, 34
  metastatic. *See* Metastatic
    carcinoma
Neoplastic-appearing erythroblasts,
    49
Neuroblastoma, metastasis of, 133
Neutropenia
  chronic idiopathic, 64
  cyclic, granulocytic hypoplasia
    in, 65
  in preleukemic state, 73
Neutrophilia
  from cortisone, 64
  in preleukemic state, 73
  pseudoneutrophilia, 64
Newborn, marrow in, 19
  hemosiderin in, 56
  hypercellular, 25
Niemann-Pick disease
  ceroid-containing histiocytes in,
    144, 146
  foam cells in, 142
Nodules
  lymphoid. *See* Lymphoid nodules
  siderofibrotic, 160, 161

Normoblasts, 41–42
  compared to lymphocytes, 41, 95,
    96
  compared to megaloblasts, 46, 47
  macronormoblasts, 43, 47
  perinuclear halo in, 41, 43
  in thalassemia, 58

Orotic acid aciduria, megaloblastosis
    in, 48
Osteitis fibrosa, 196–197
Osteoblasts
  in osteomalacia, 195
  in Paget's disease, 198
Osteoclasts, 27, 31
  in osteitis fibrosa, 196
  in Paget's disease, 197–198
Osteoid seam
  in osteitis fibrosa, 196, 197
  in osteomalacia, 194, 195
Osteomalacia, 194–195
Osteopenia, in metastatic tumors,
    139
Osteoporosis, 191, 194
  mast cells in, 92, 194
Osteosclerosis, 191
  in metastatic tumors, 139
  with myelofibrosis, 154, 191

Paget's disease, 197–199
Paramyloidosis, 85
  differential diagnosis of, 125
Parasitic infestation, eosinophilia
    in, 89
Pelger-Huët cells, 60
Periarteritis nodosa, 183
  eosinophilia in, 89
  plasma cells in, 78
Periodic acid–Schiff reaction,
    212–213
Peripheral smears, examination of,
    15–16
Pigments in marrow, 180
Plasma cells, 75–88
  ceroid-containing histiocytes with,
    146
  decreased, 77
  distribution of, 77
  in eosinophilic fibrohistiocytic
    lesion, 174
  flaming, 77
  with Gaucher's cells, 148, 149
  in heavy-chain disease, 88